The Adventures of Fuzzy the Virus

Helping Children Understand the COVID Pandemic

"It's going to be OK!"

Fuzzy the Virus tells the story of the coronavirus pandemic... in a safe and optimistic way that child psychologists believe help children better understand and cope with their own existential anxieties and dilemmas.

Fuzzy the Virus is a fairly tale of sorts, as told through the adventures and world-wide travels of the virus itself. It is a story that, ultimately, is about survival and human optimism... Fuzzy the Virus is a belief that 'It's going to be OK'... that we can all learn, grow, and overcome our scary challenges.

The Adventures of Fuzzy the Virus
Helping Children Understand the COVID Pandemic
ISBN: 9798760659309
Written by Russ Hafferkamp
Illustrated by Alex Andriesse.

Copyright: ©2021 and Trademark Protected: Fuzzy the Virus™. All rights reserved by Russ Hafferkamp Printed in the United States of America. No part of this book may be used, reproduced, or transmitted in whole or in part, in any manner or by any means whatsoever, without permission of the author.

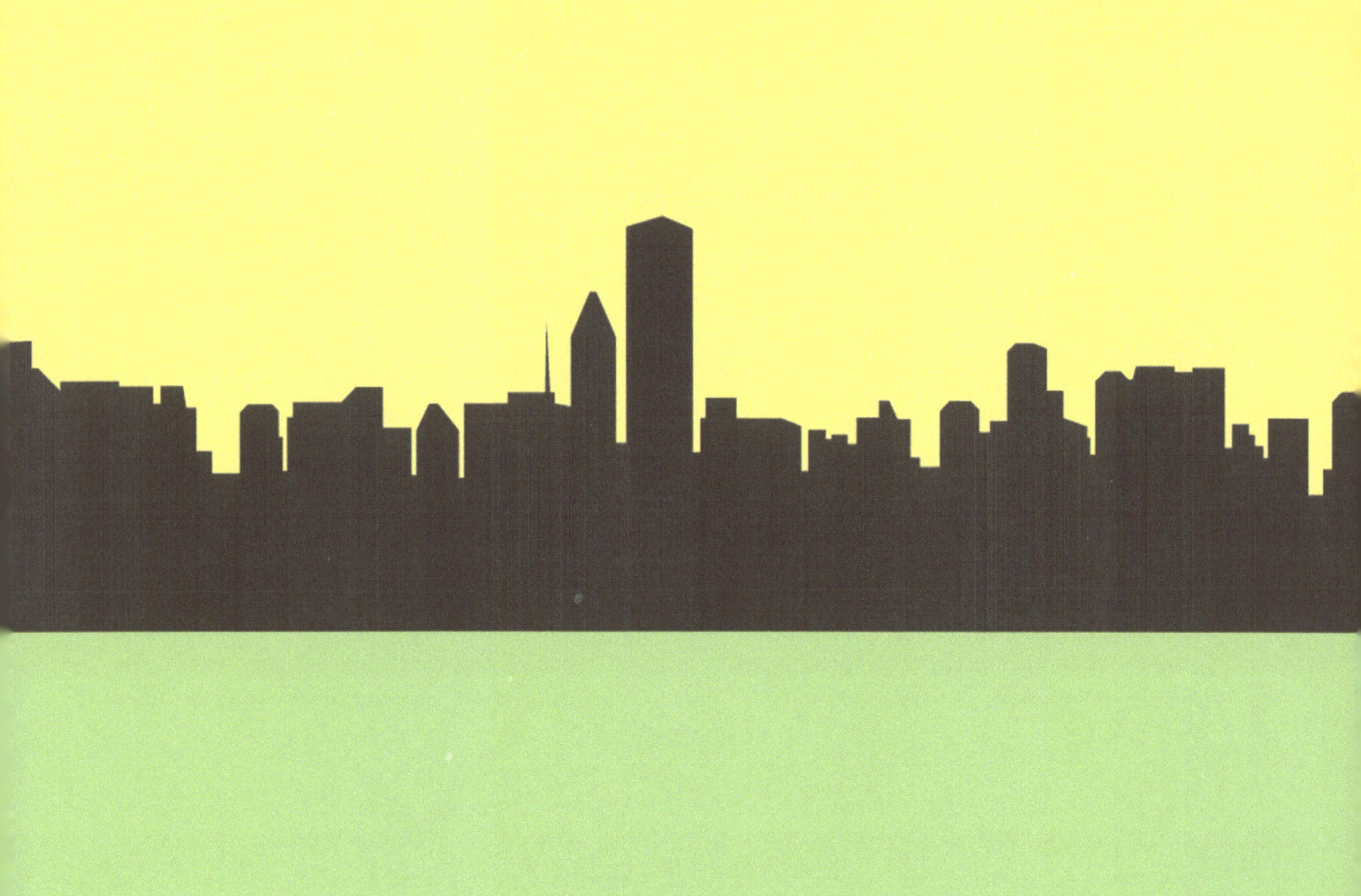

This is Fuzzy.
    Nobody really knows who Fuzzy is... or where he was born.
Nobody really even knows if Fuzzy is a he, or a she... or maybe even both!
    But nobody really cares.

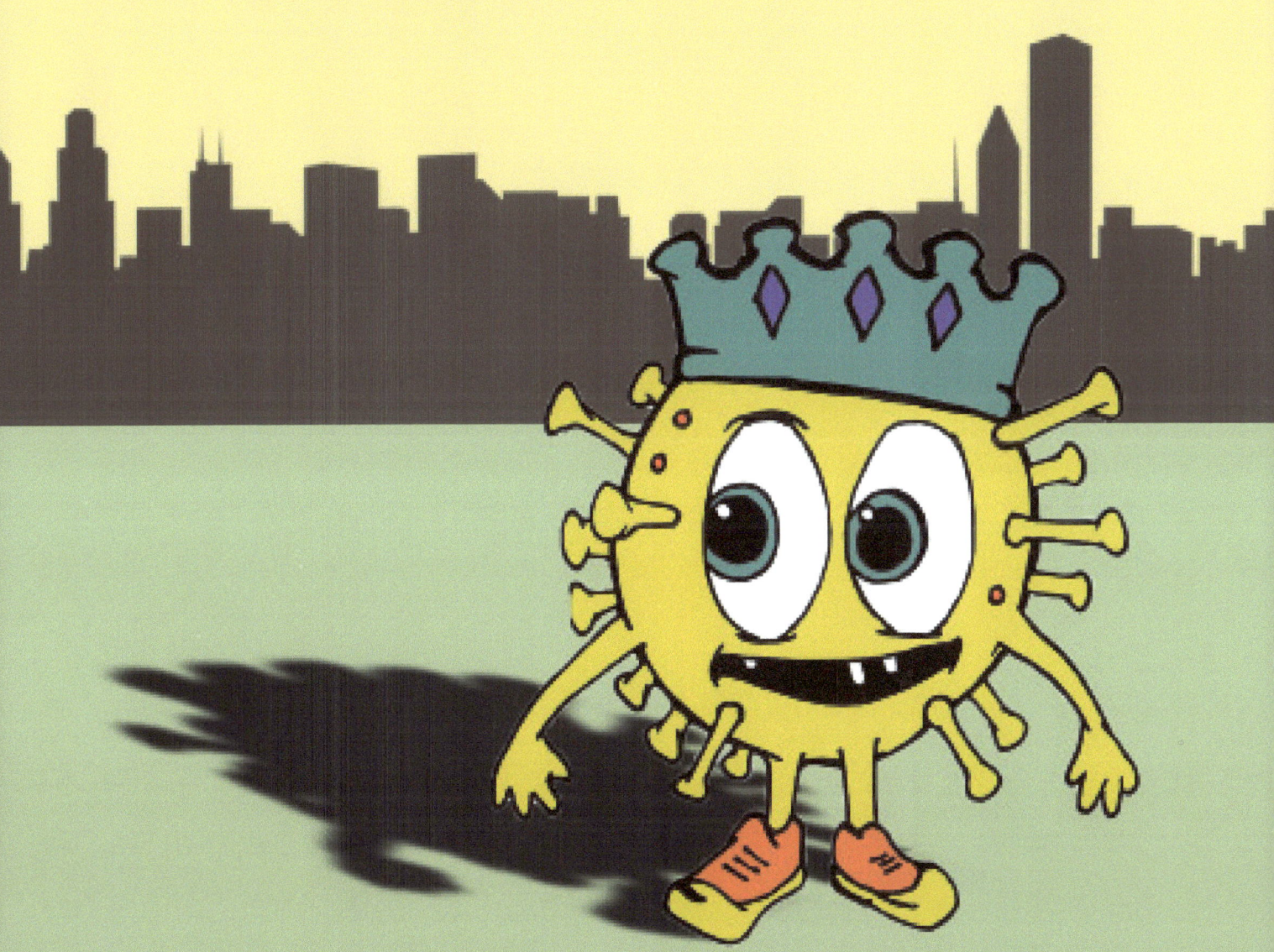

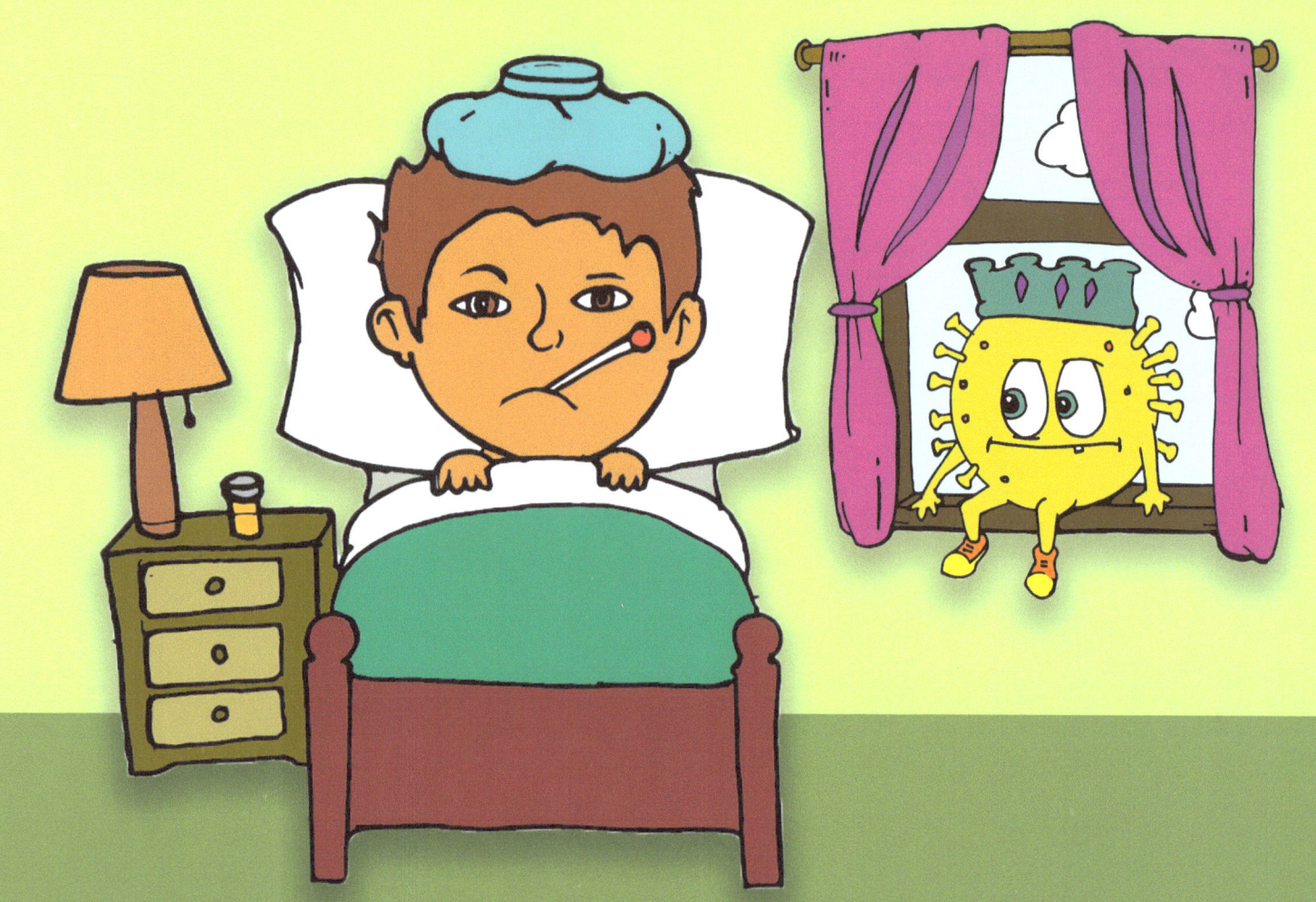

You see, Fuzzy is a virus and viruses are very scary.
 A virus can cause humans to get sick... like the flu... chicken pox... or even the sniffles you get from a cold.
Some viruses are extra mean and strong!
 If you're not careful, some viruses can even put you in the hospital... or worse!

That's why parents are always saying...

"Be sure to wash your hands!"

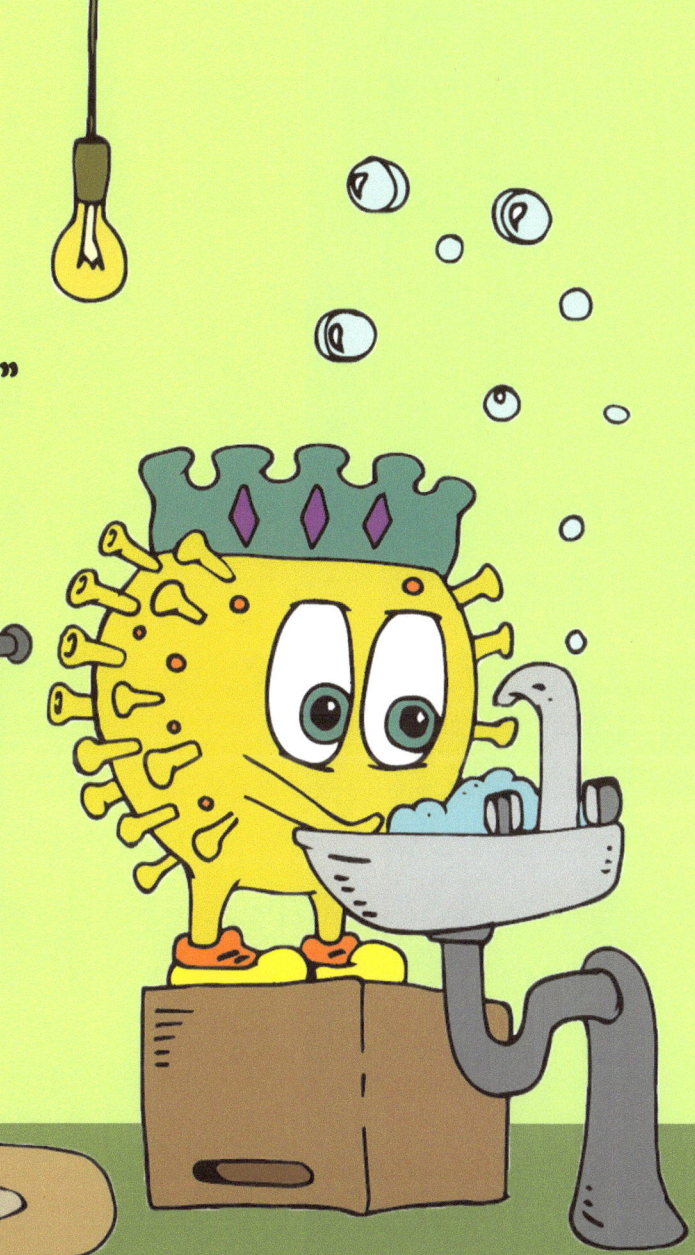

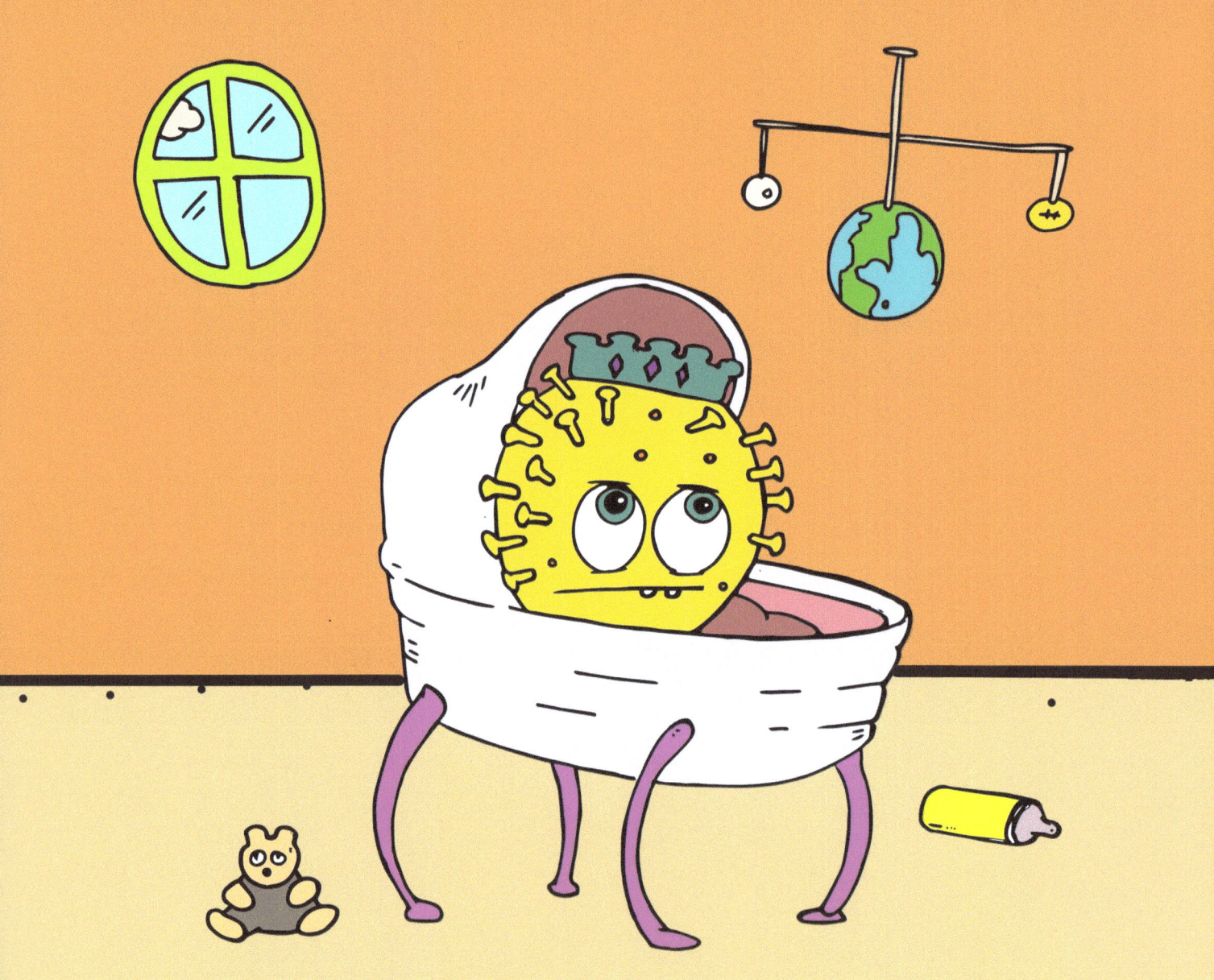

Every virus is born to travel the globe, to explore and spread far and wide... and Fuzzy was no different.

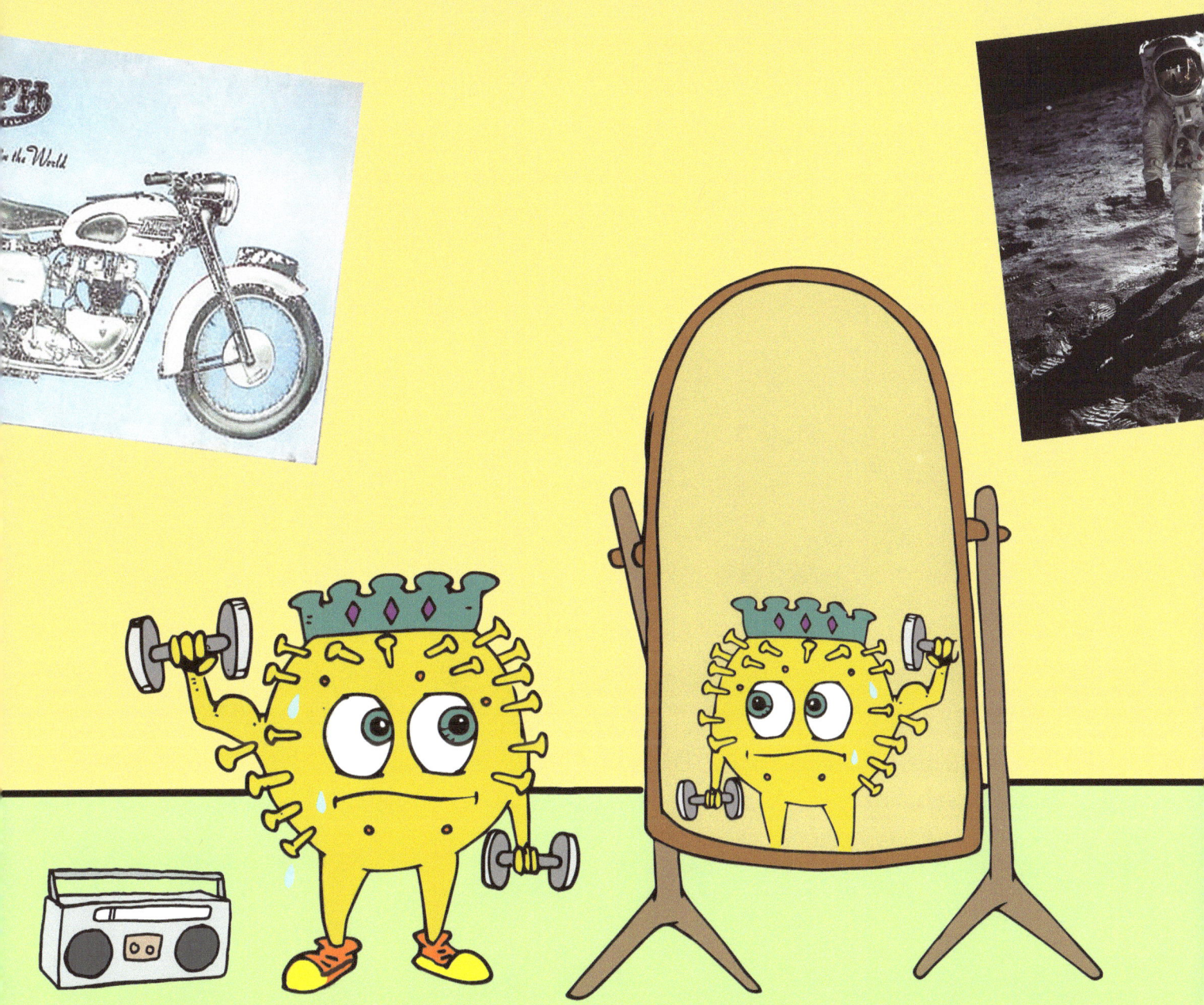

His parents always encouraged Fuzzy to be strong and independent. When he was old enough and strong enough, he was ready to begin his adventure.

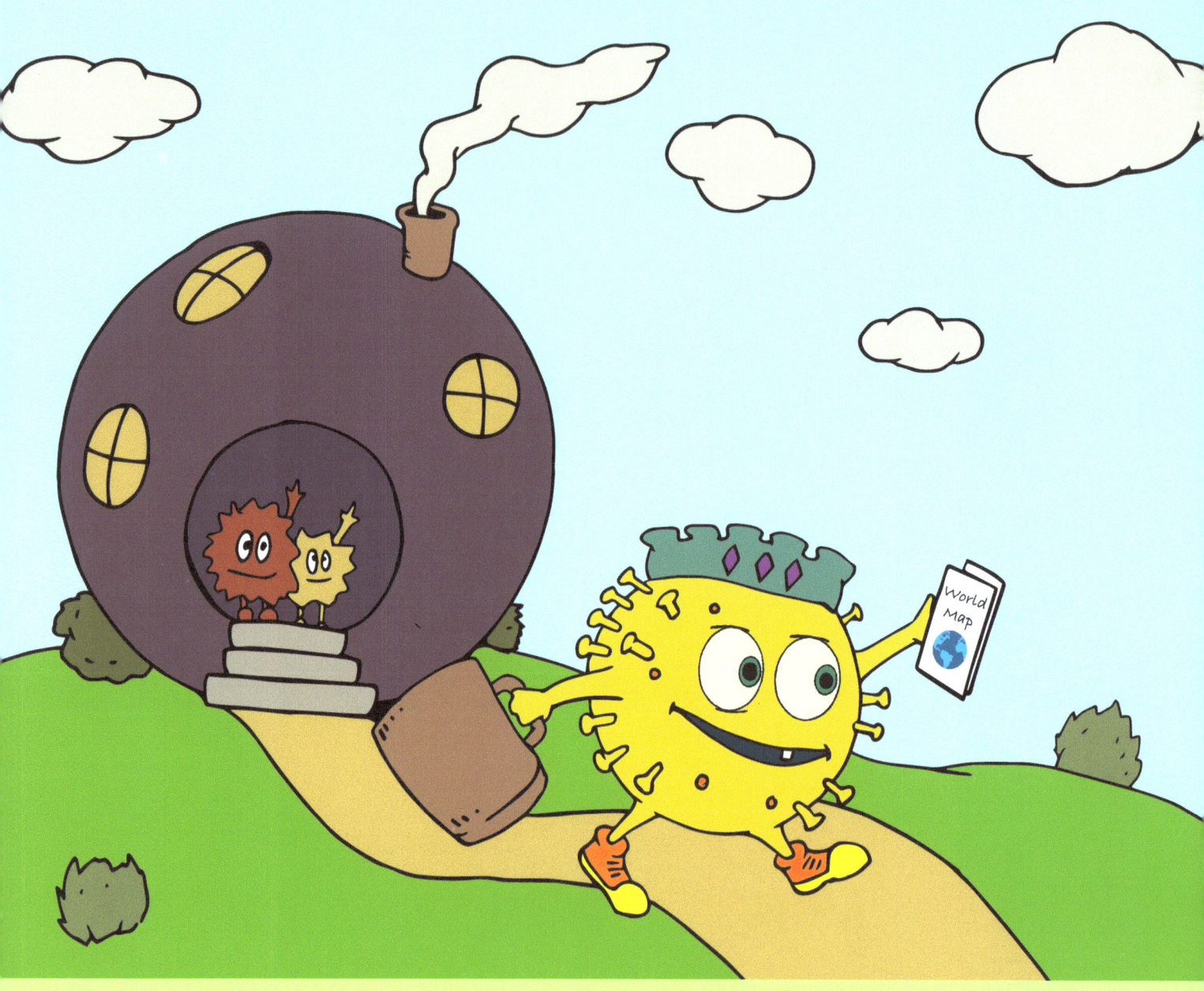

He was so excited to meet many different people, from many different countries... but Fuzzy would soon find out that the world was not ready to welcome him as their friend.

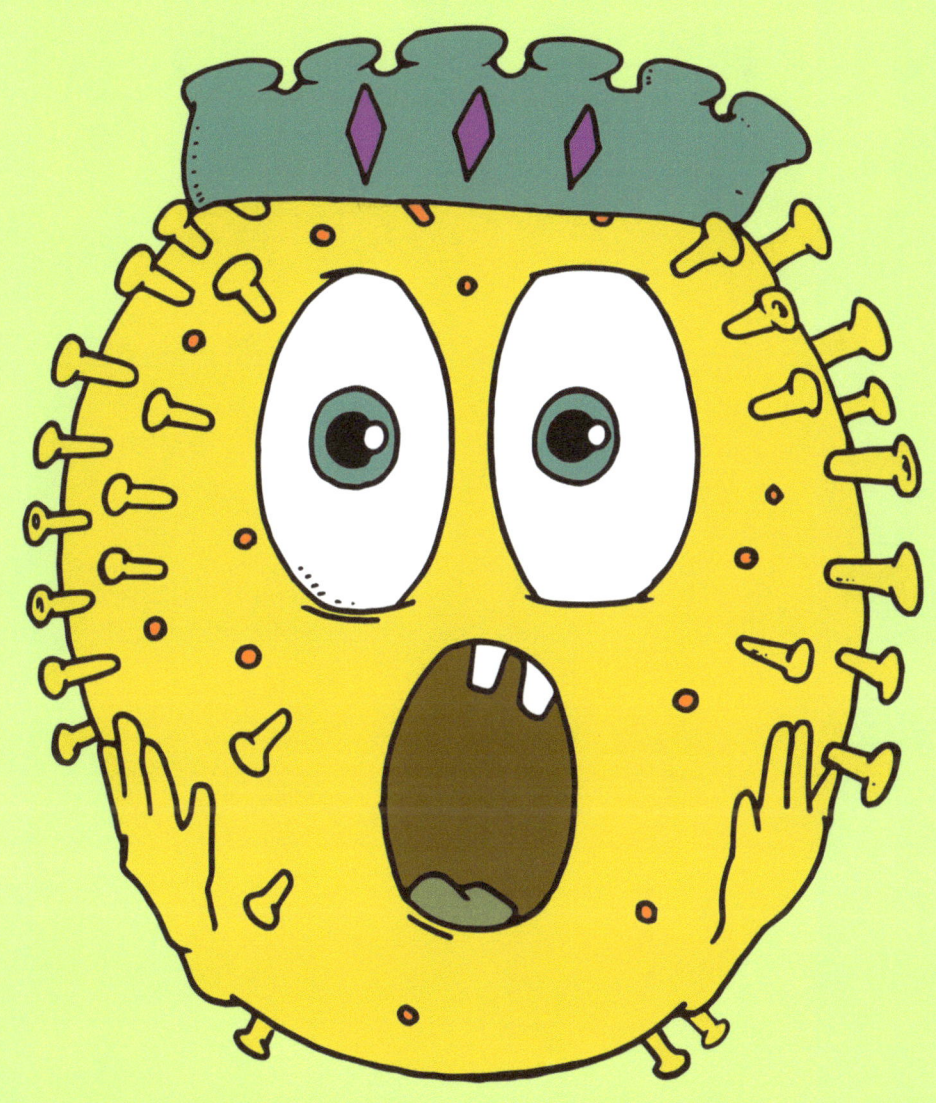

You see Fuzzy did not realize he was a virus. His parents never told him.

Uh-oh!

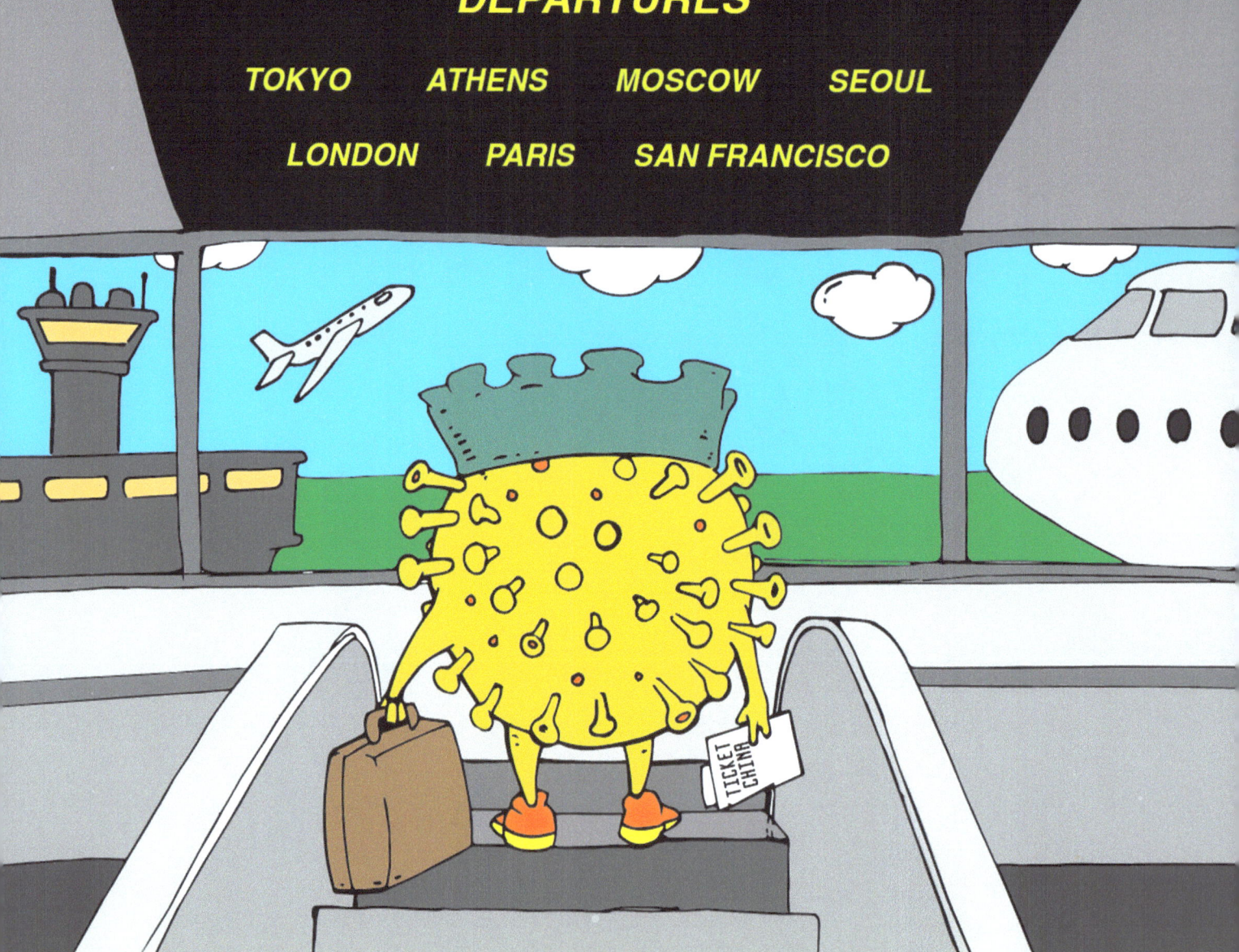

One day when the world was too busy to notice, Fuzzy started out on his adventure. He visited China and made gobs of new friends. He was thrilled!

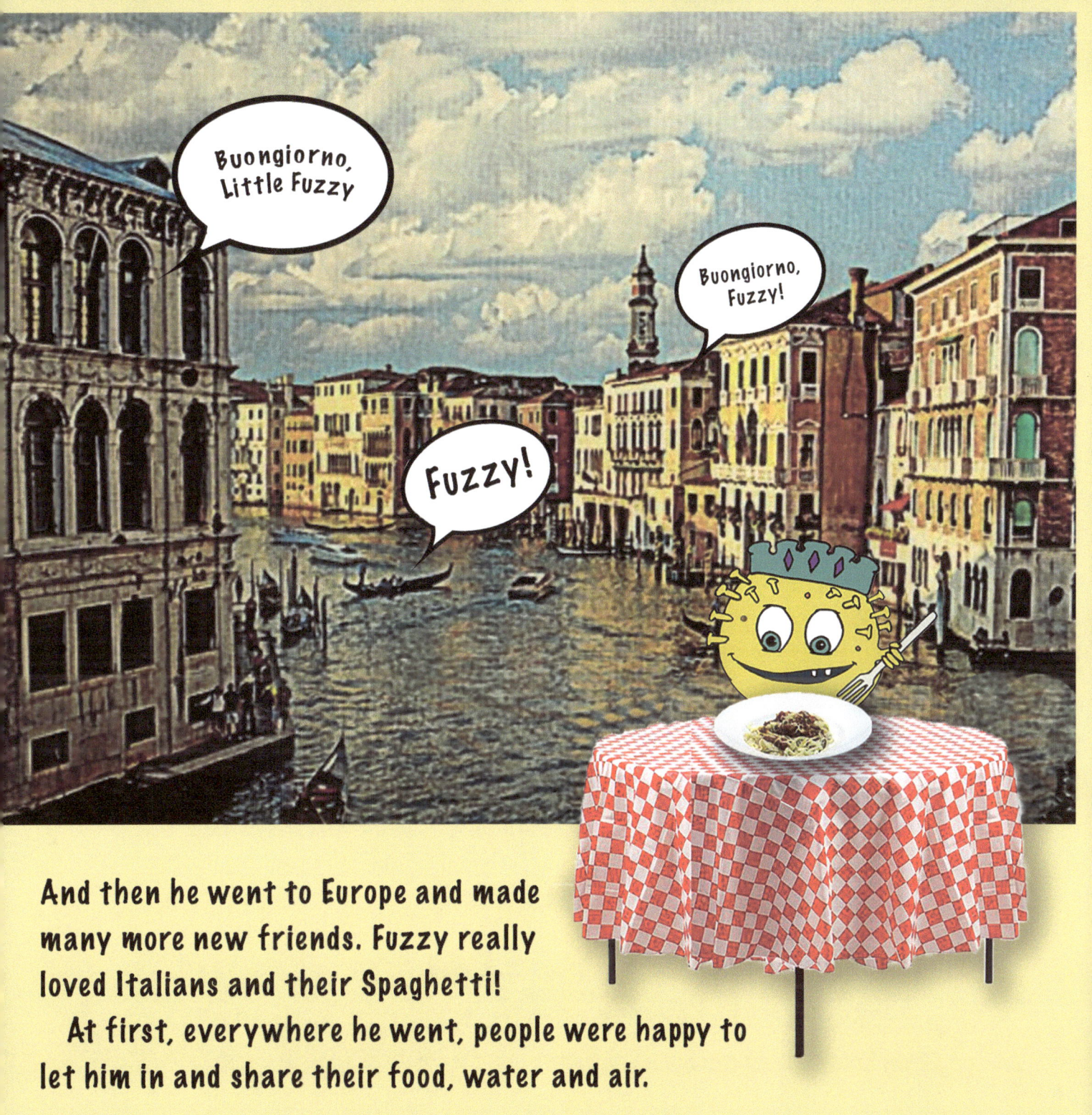

And then he went to Europe and made many more new friends. Fuzzy really loved Italians and their Spaghetti!

At first, everywhere he went, people were happy to let him in and share their food, water and air.

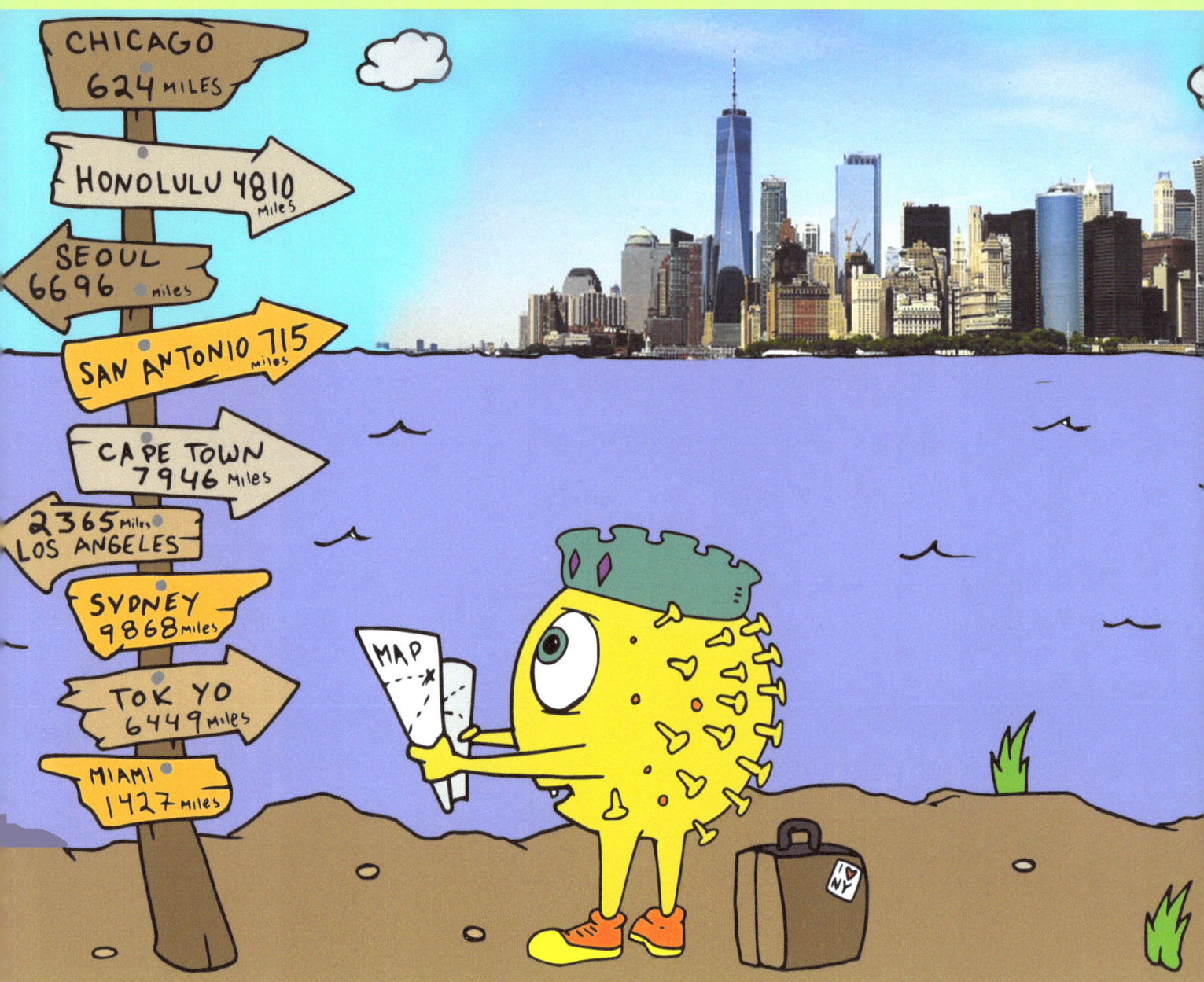

Fuzzy was having so much fun he decided to go to New York City, and then visit everywhere in the United States and then over to Africa and Australia and even Japan and Korea!

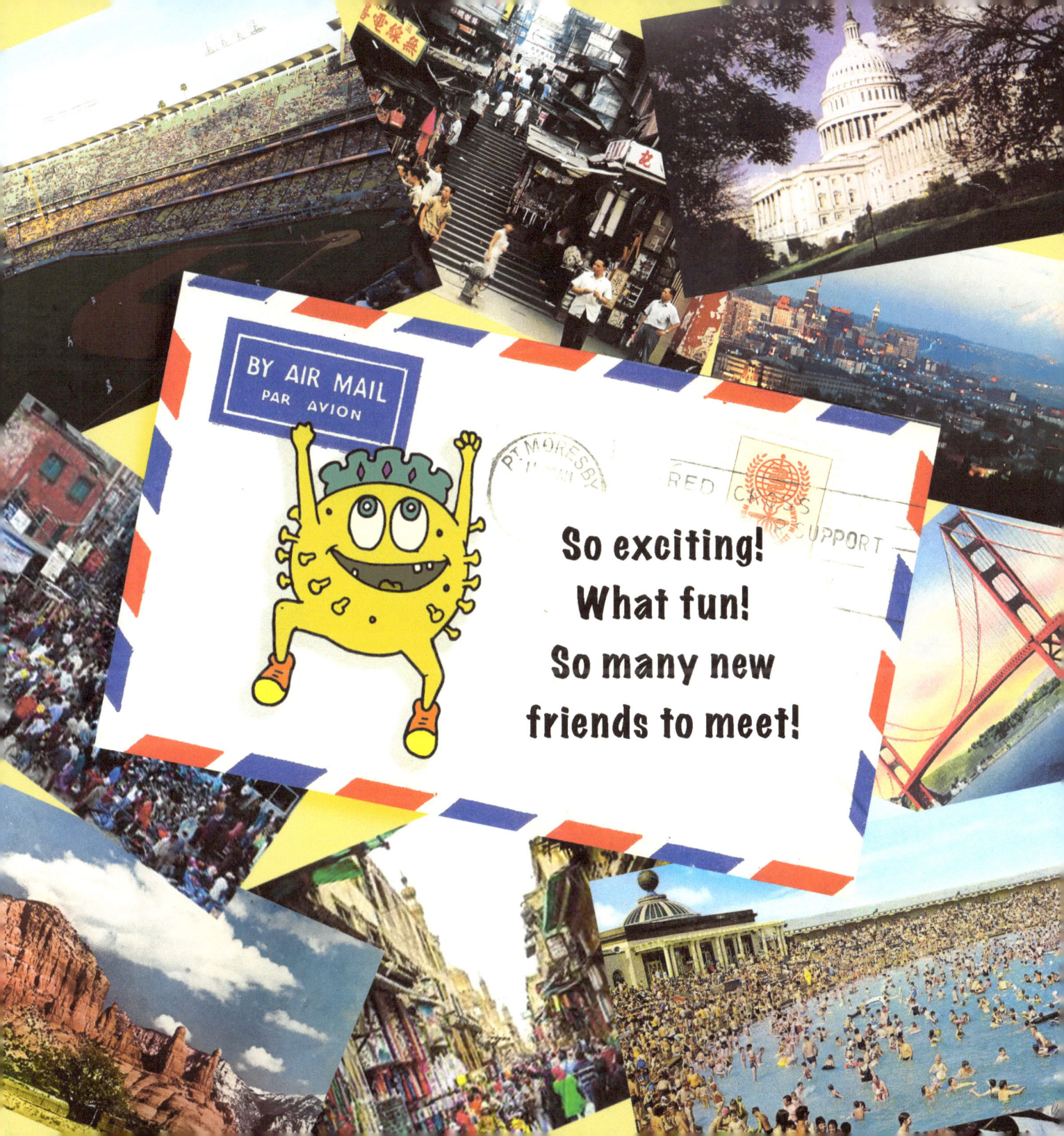

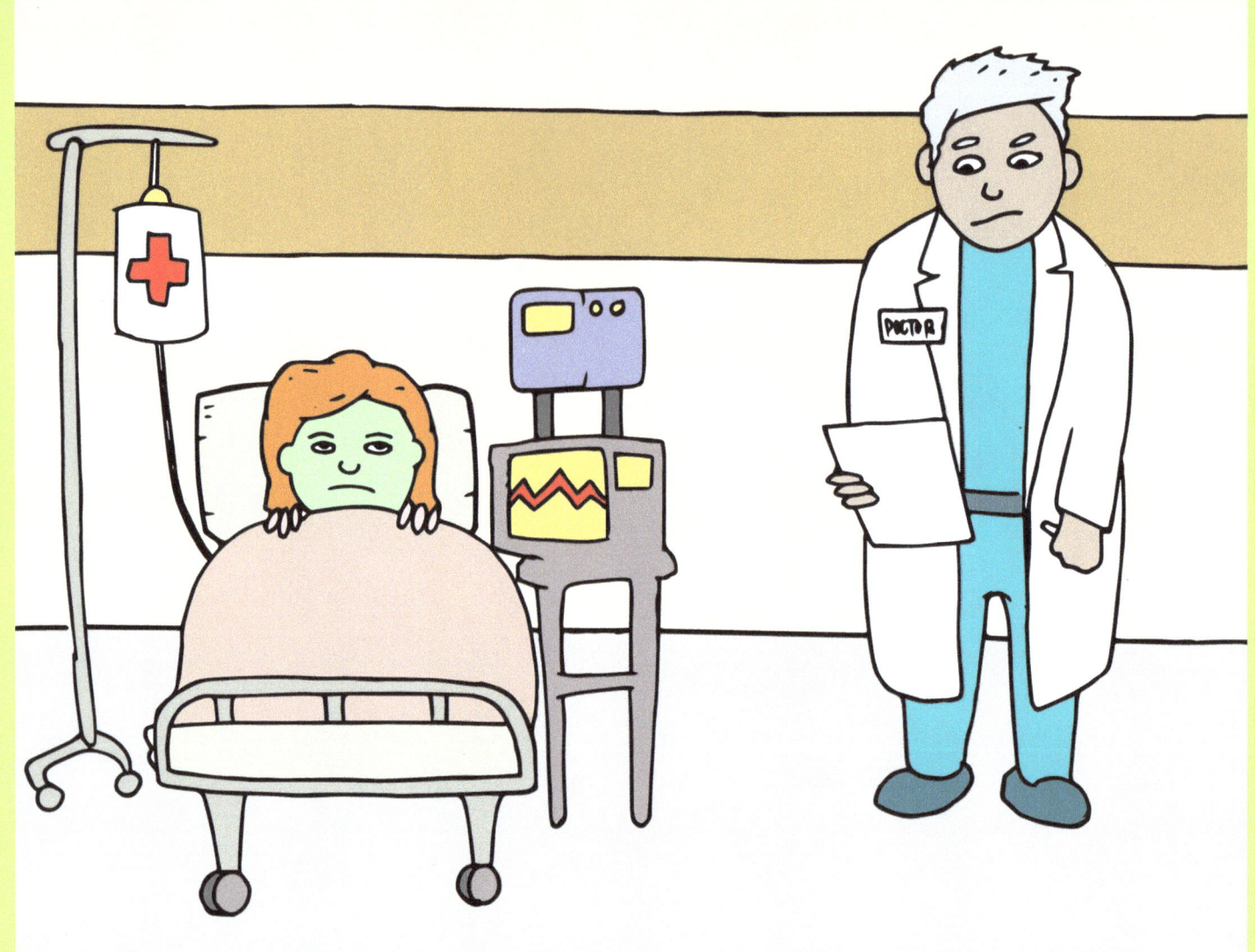

But then something very scary began to happen...
   Fuzzy's new friends all began to get sick.
They coughed and had sore throats and even had a temperature!
   Some got so sick they had to go to the hospital. The doctors
   and nurses were very brave, and they tried very hard to help
   all the sick people!

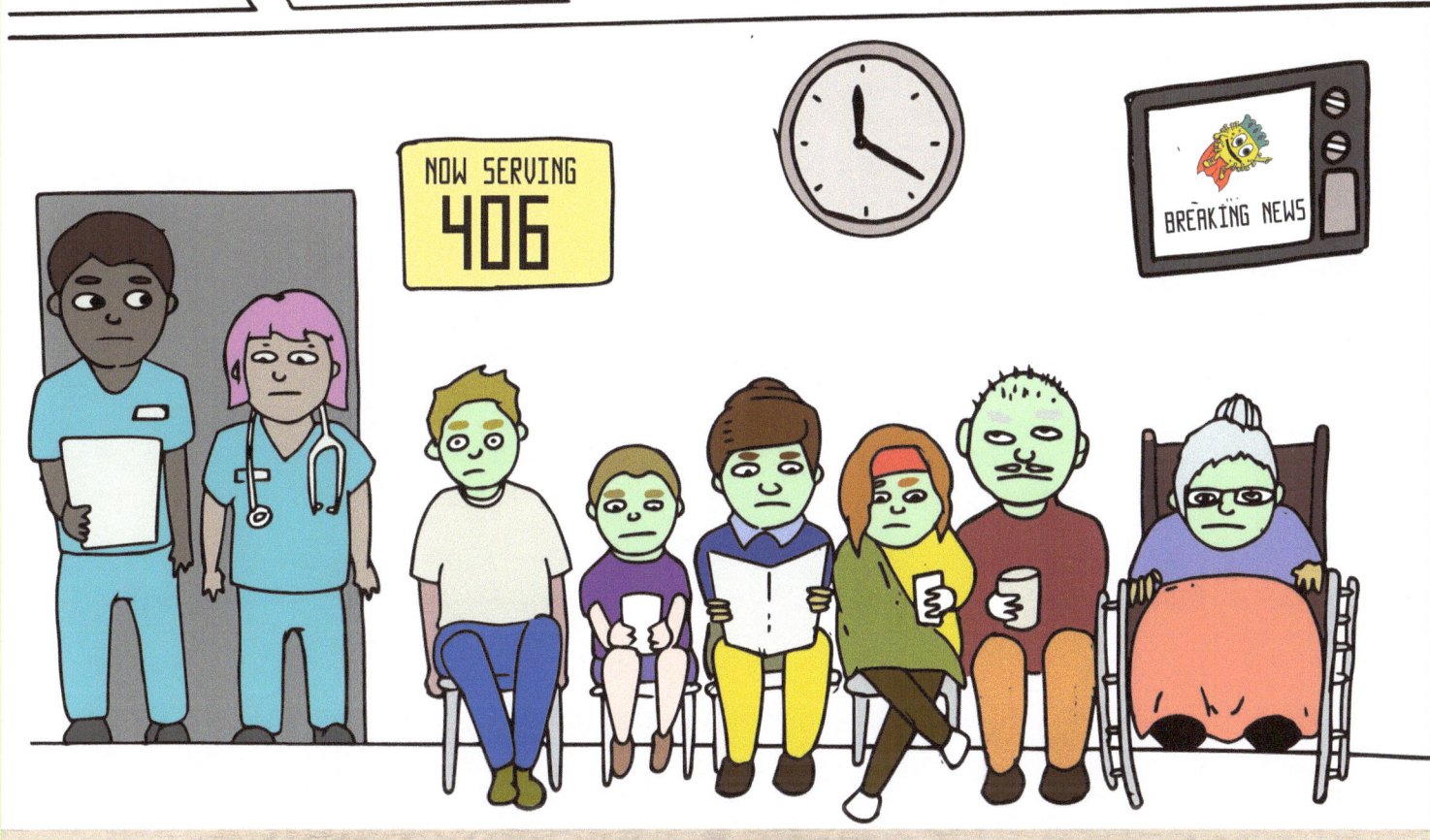

But there were so many.
 Some people just couldn't be helped, and it was a sad day when that happened.

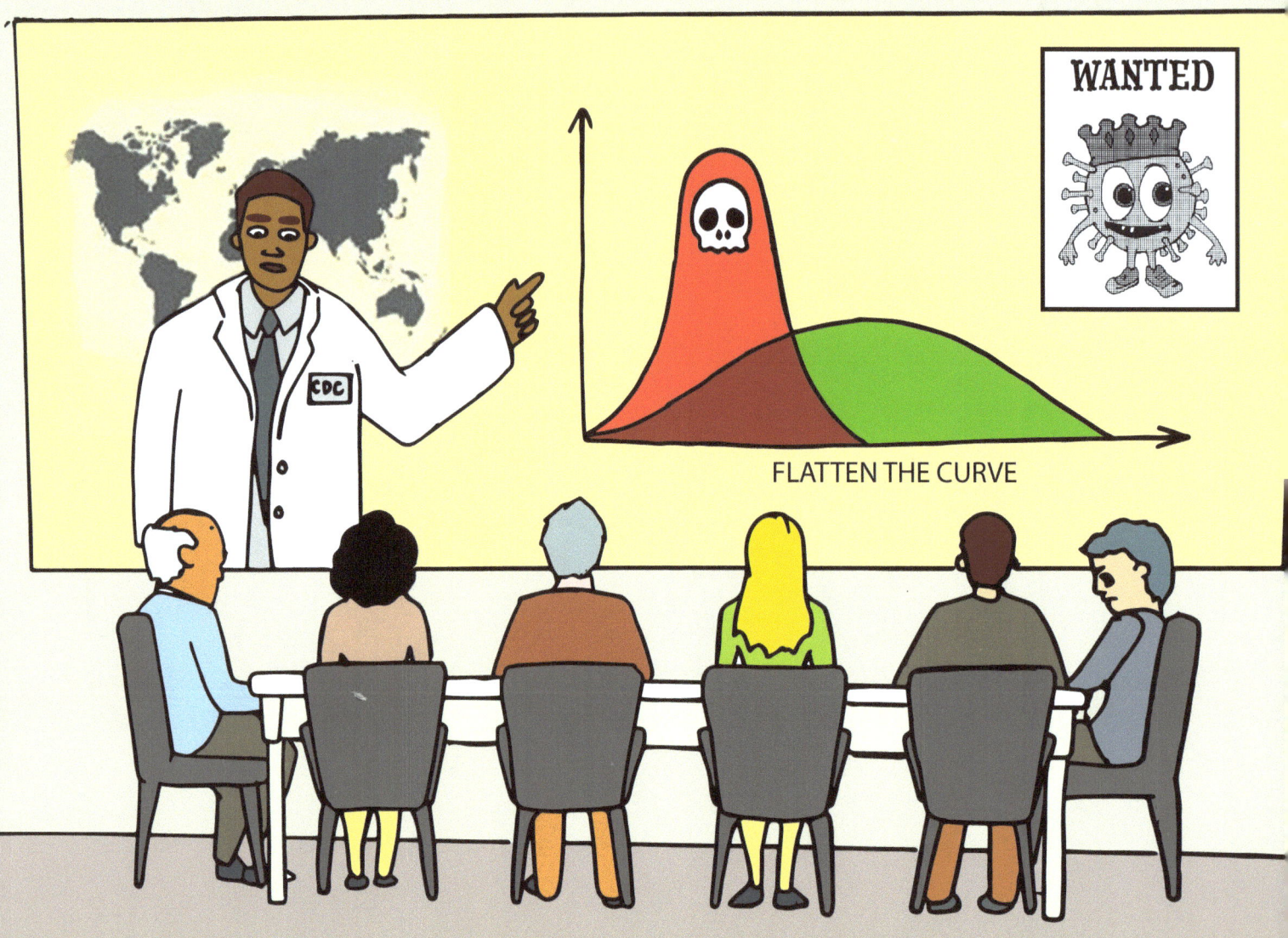

Something had to be done... and done quickly!

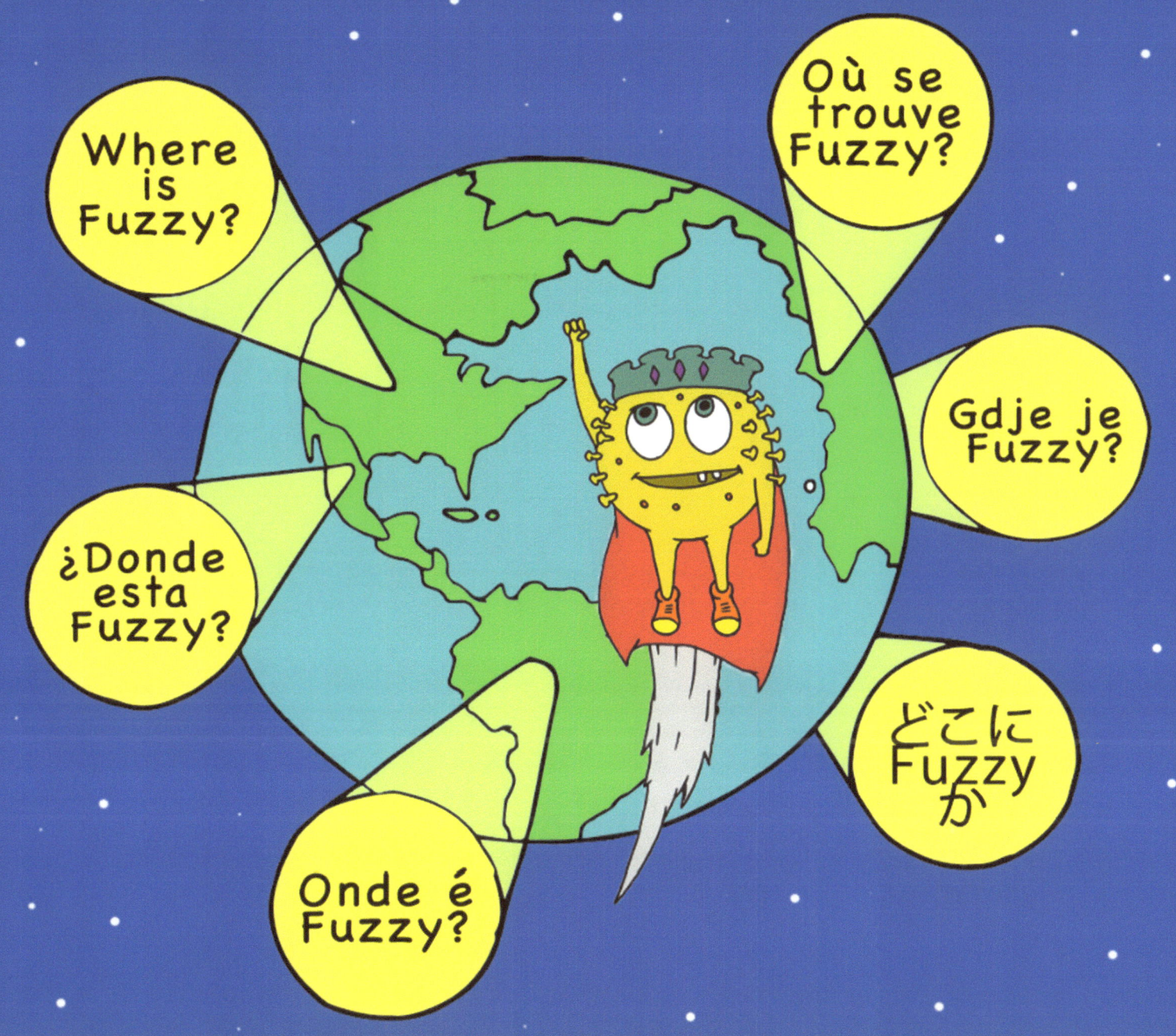

Everybody in the whole-wide-world became very afraid of Fuzzy.
Everyone was asking "Where is Fuzzy now?"
Nobody knew where he was. They looked for him everywhere.

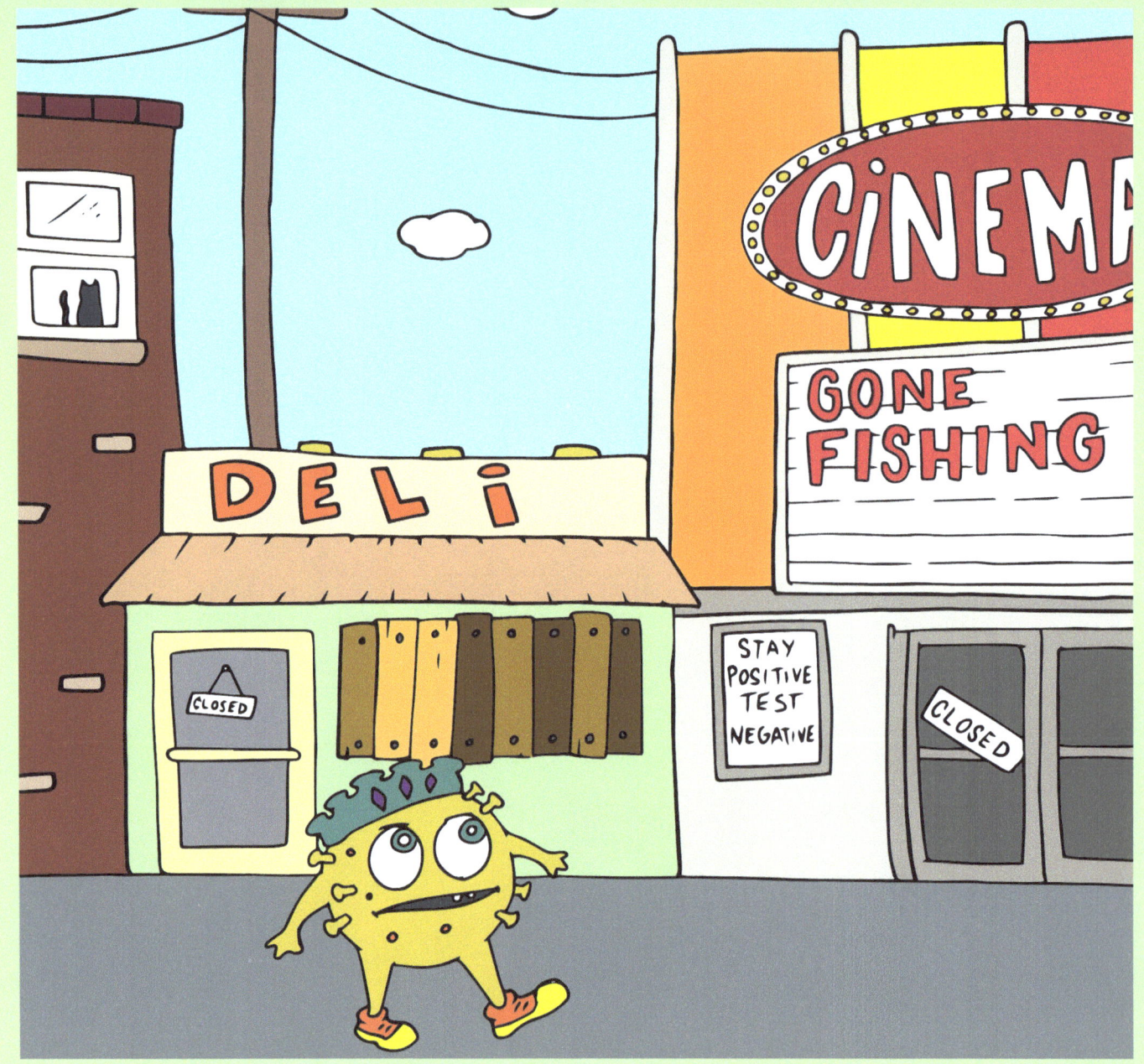

Everyone began staying home and hiding from Fuzzy. Soon all the stores and movies and restaurants began to close down. Even the schools closed their doors so kids could stay home and hide from Fuzzy.

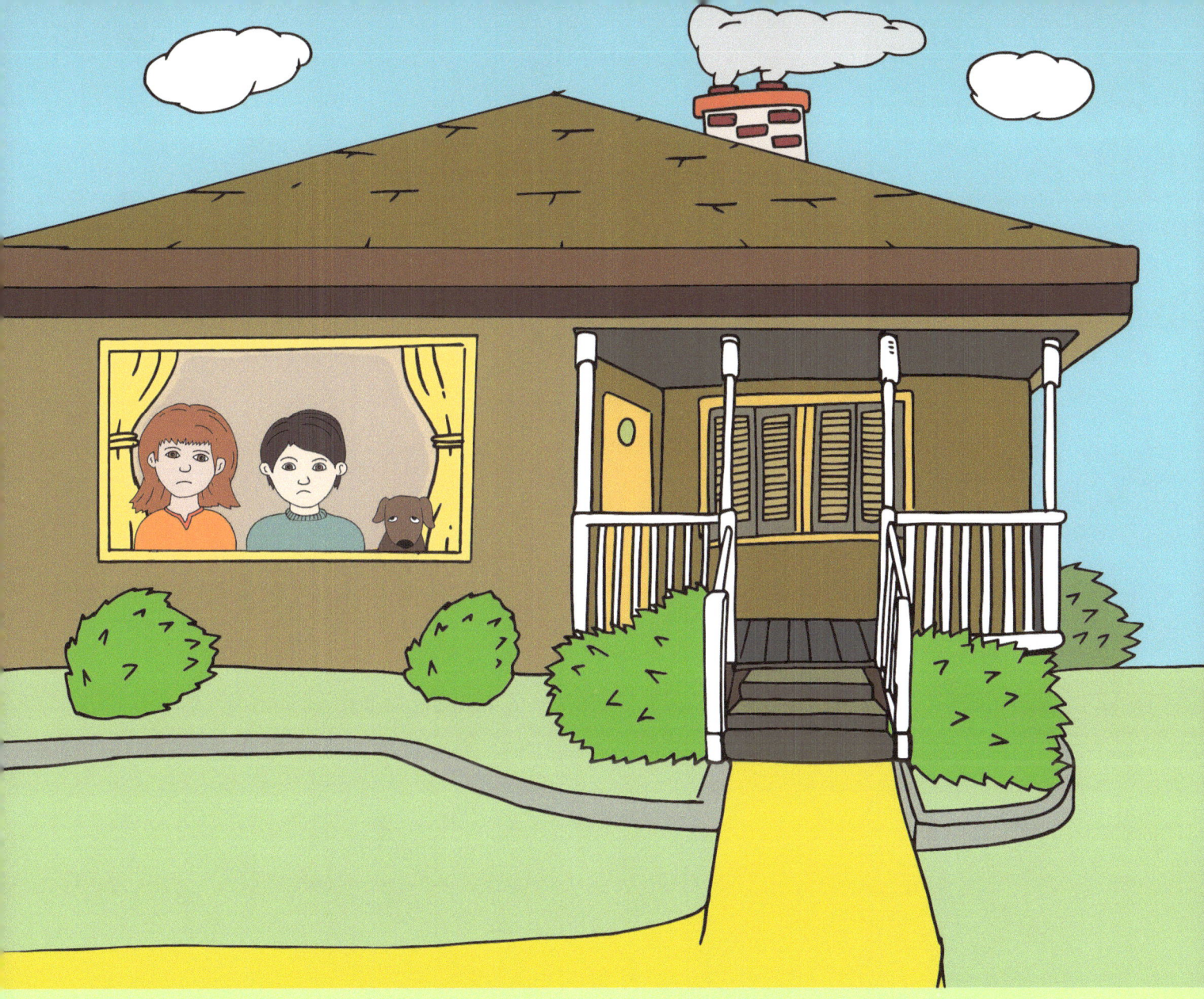

No more airplane trips or visits to the ice cream shop.
No more days at the beach, or visits to grandpa or grandma.
No more playing in the park with other kids... no more birthday parties!

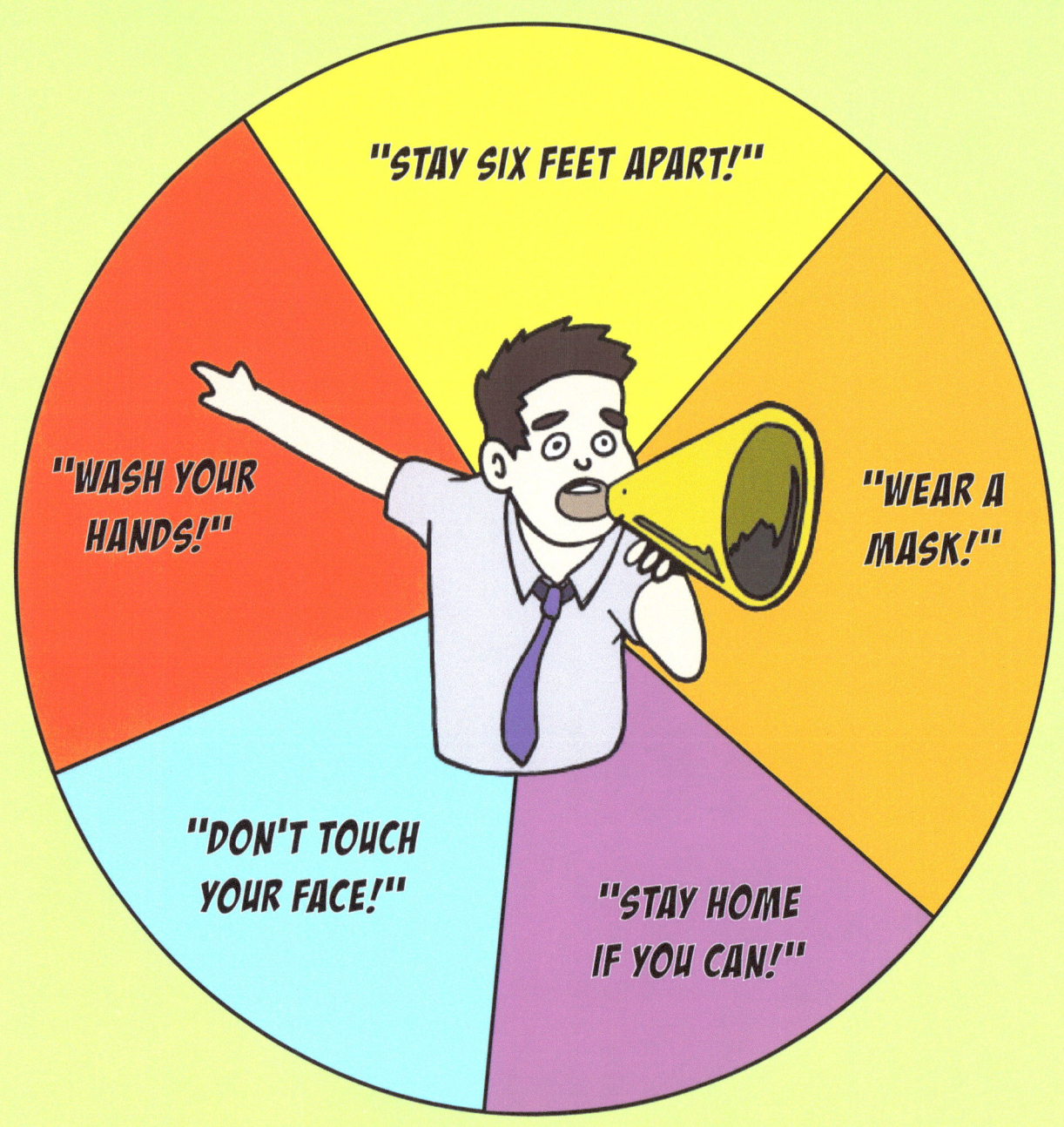

Everyone was now saying...
"Stay six feet apart!"   "Stay home if you can!"
"Wear a mask!"   "Don't touch your face!"   "Wash your hands!"

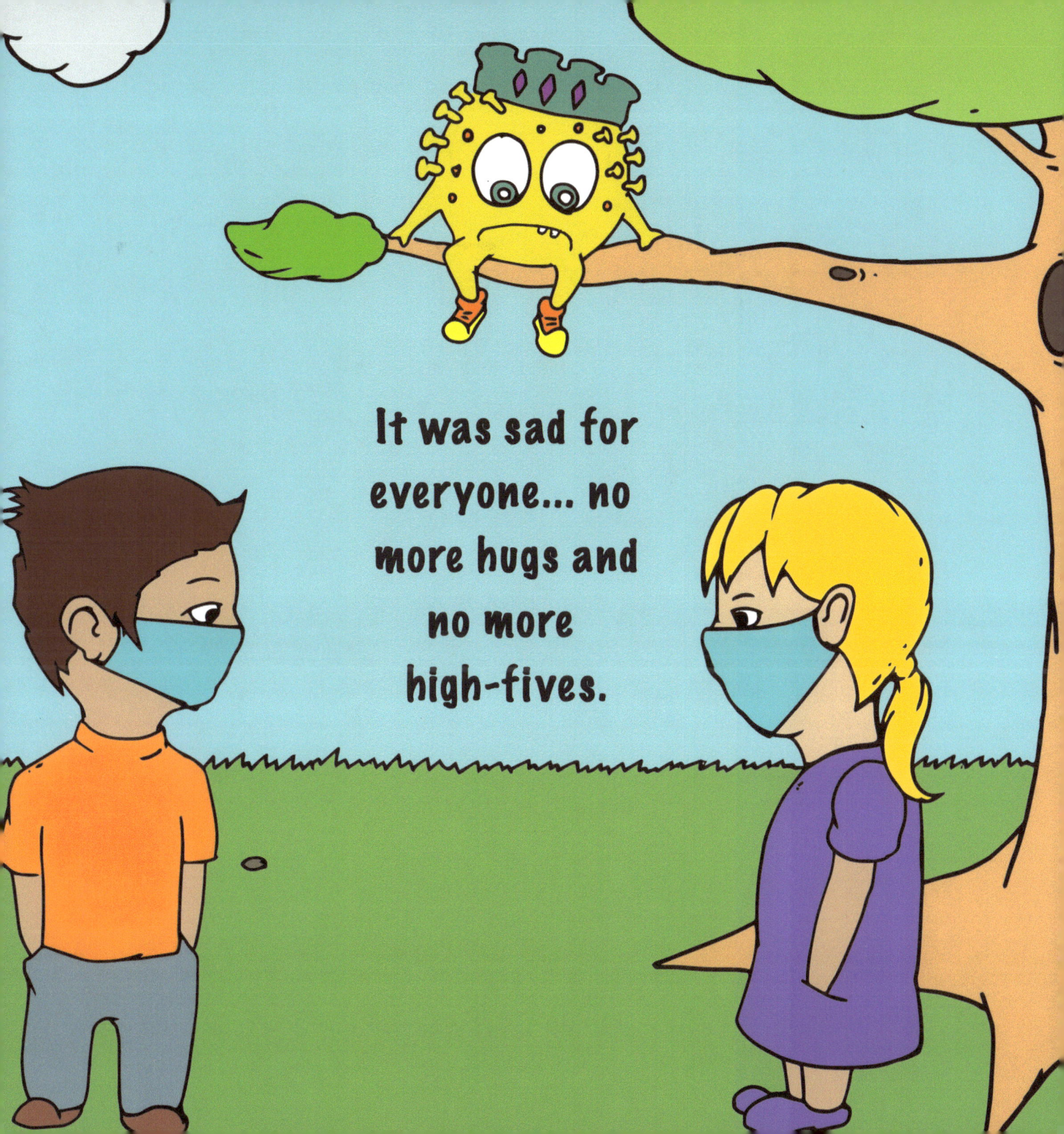

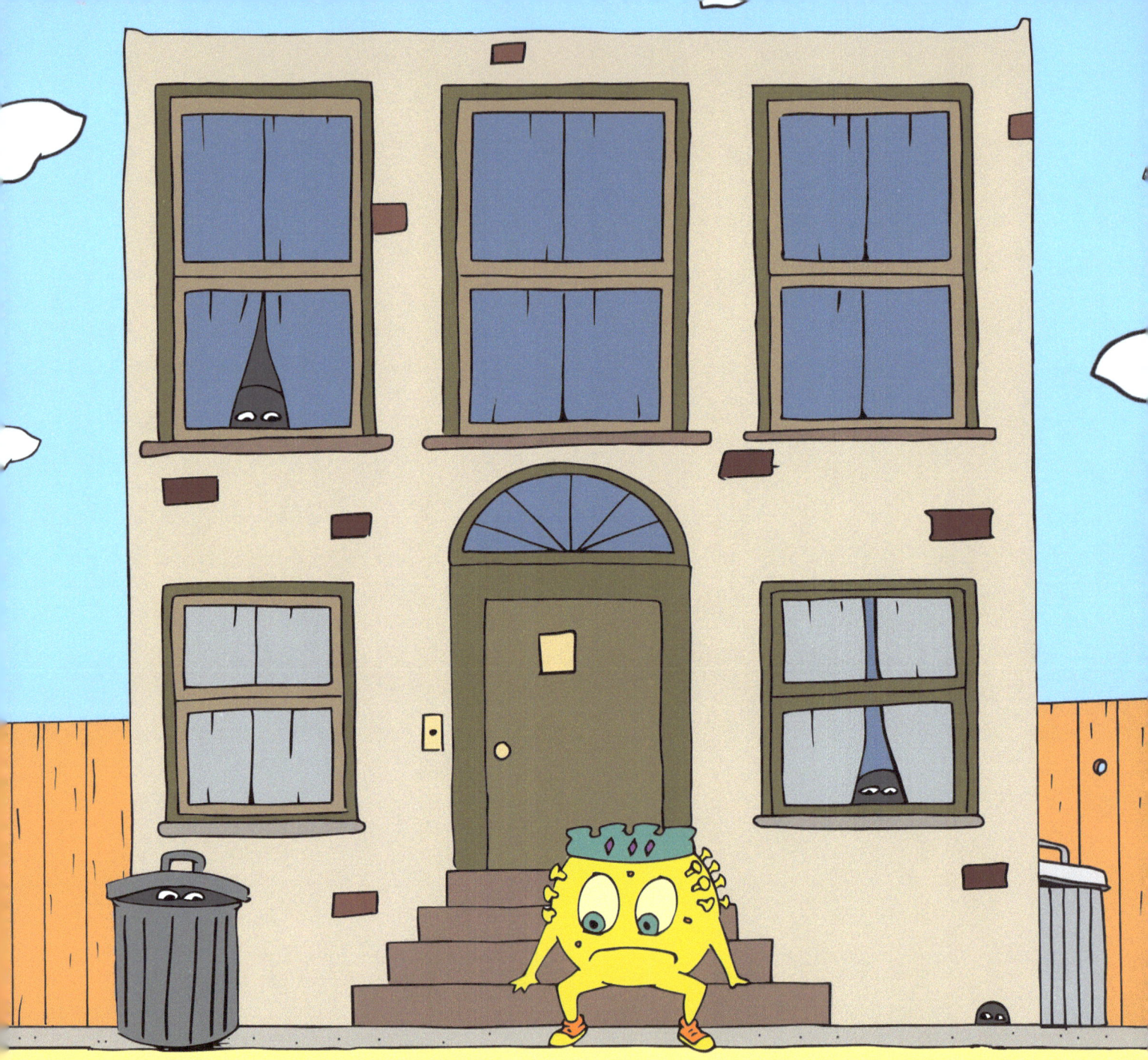

"I just want to make new friends. I just want to spread around the world like other viruses. Why is everyone so scared?" Fuzzy asked himself.

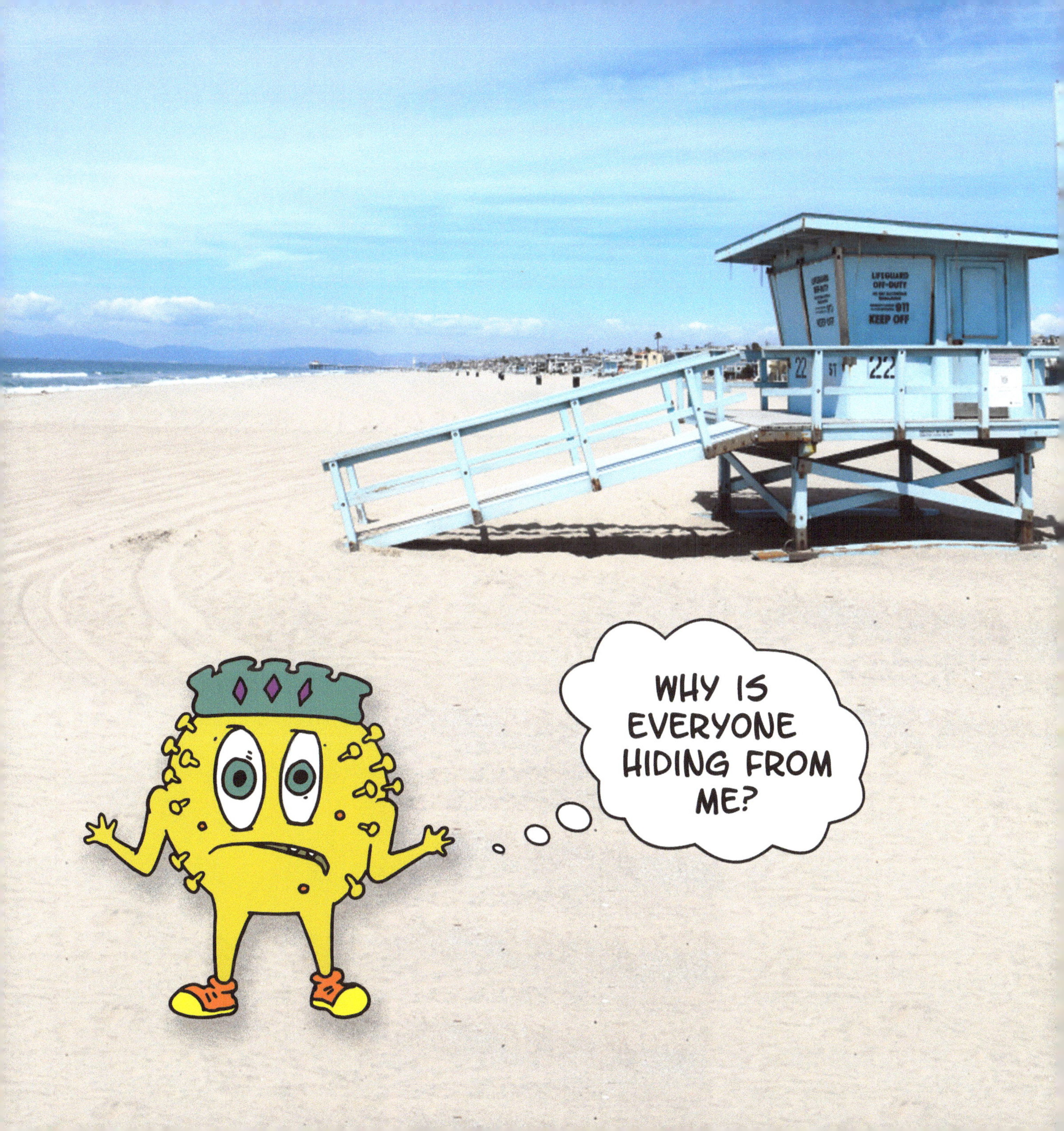

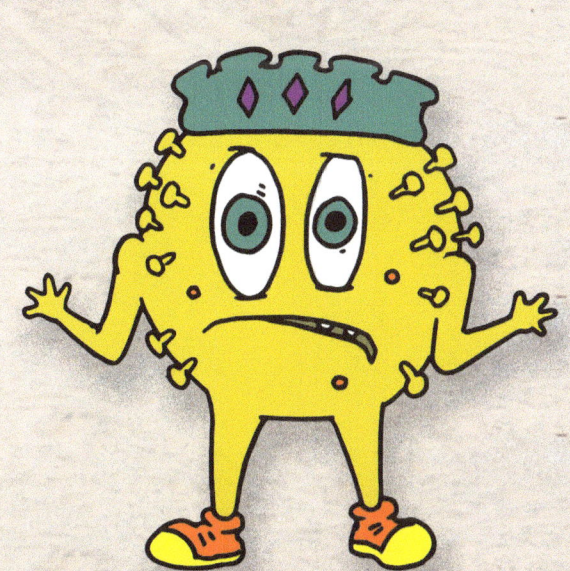

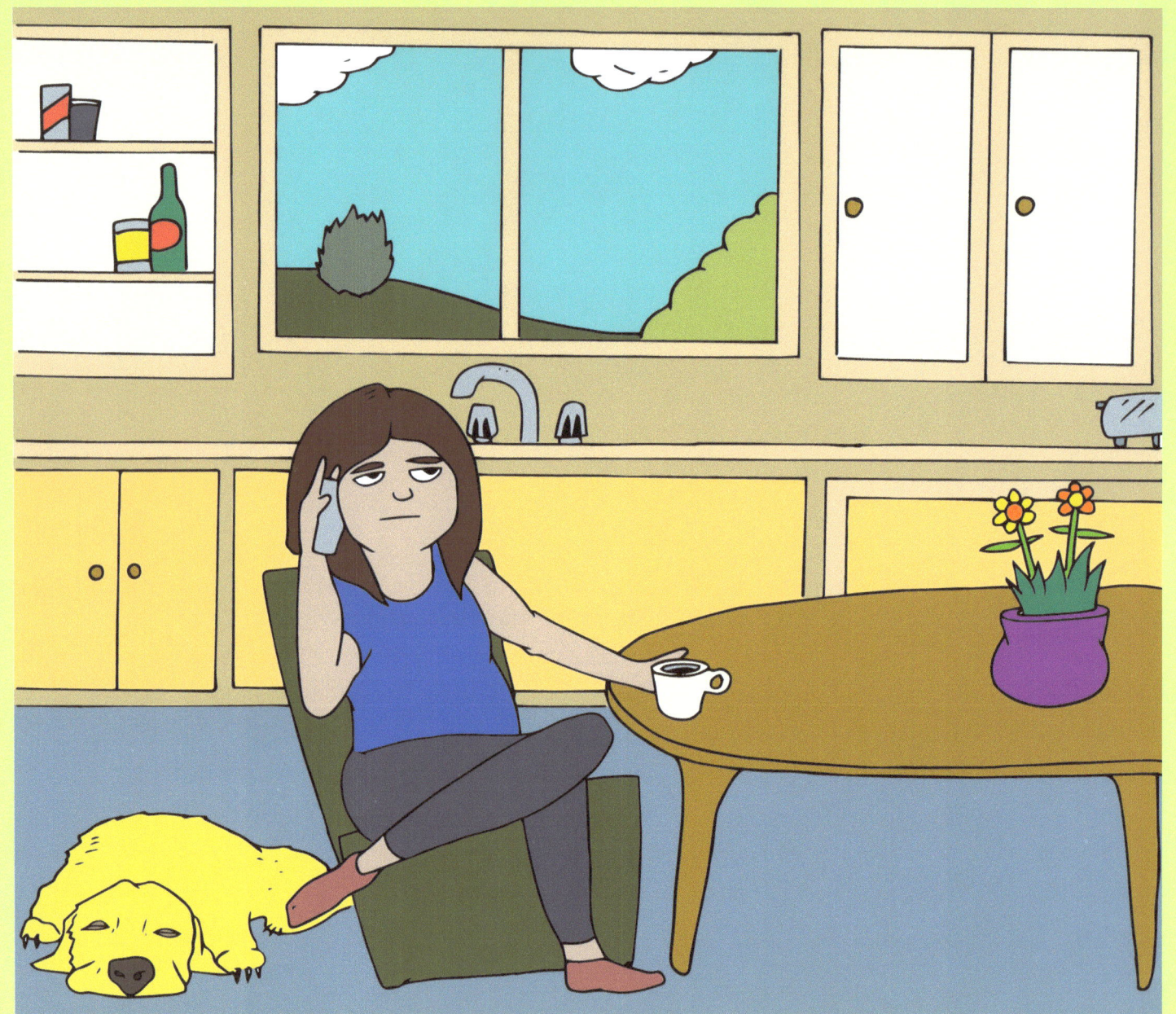

Then something very strange began to happen.
As each day passed, the world got very good at hiding from Fuzzy, and everyone got on their phones and began calling their friends and family.
"**Have you seen or heard from Fuzzy?**"

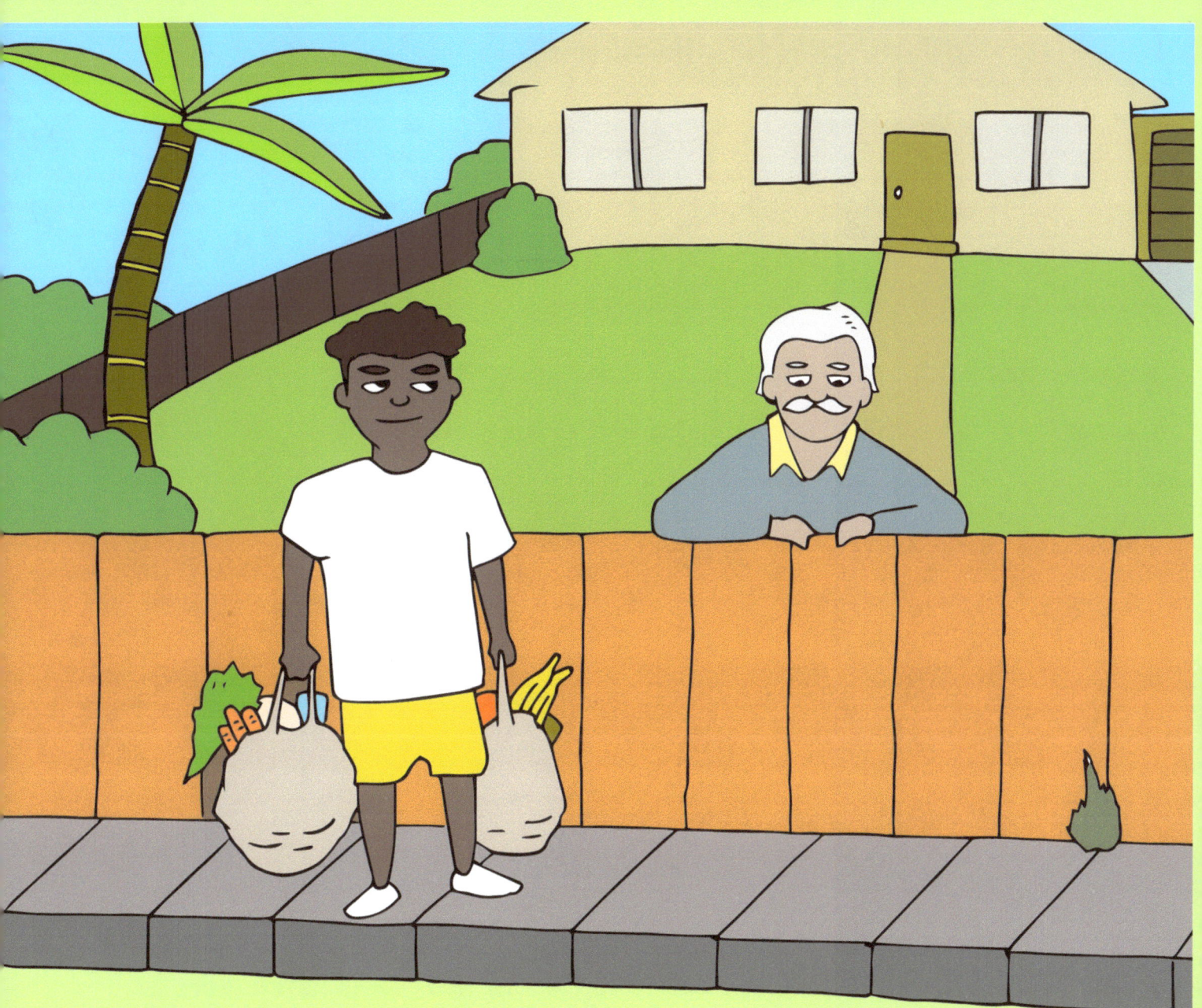

People began to call old friends and catch up on old times.
"Are you safe? How have you been? How is your family?"
People began to help and talk with their neighbors.
They would ask "Do you need anything at the store?"

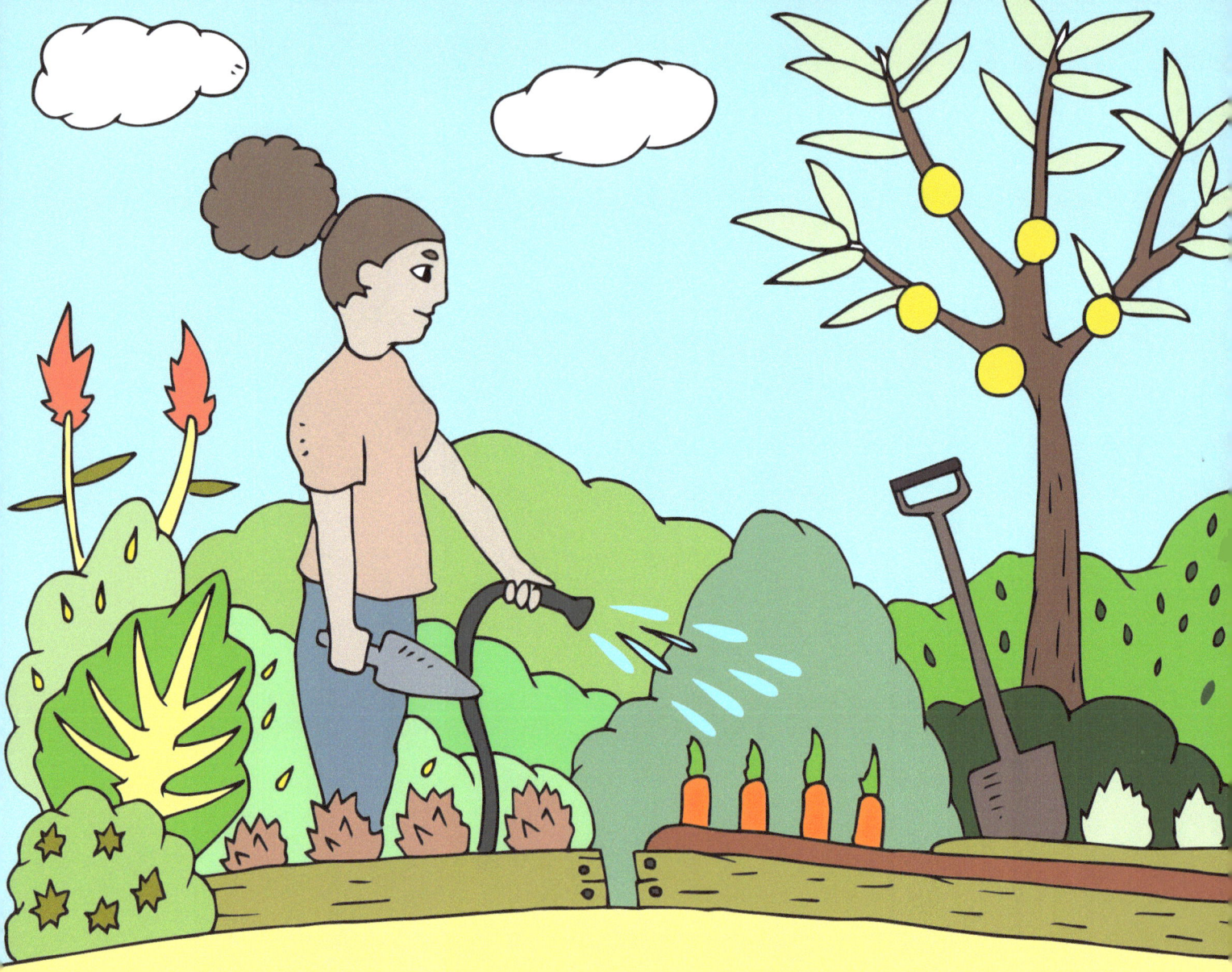

People began to share and take time to talk... and listen more... and find the time each day to just relax.

People began to become more creative... painting rocks, knitting scarfs, making jewelry and writing poetry.

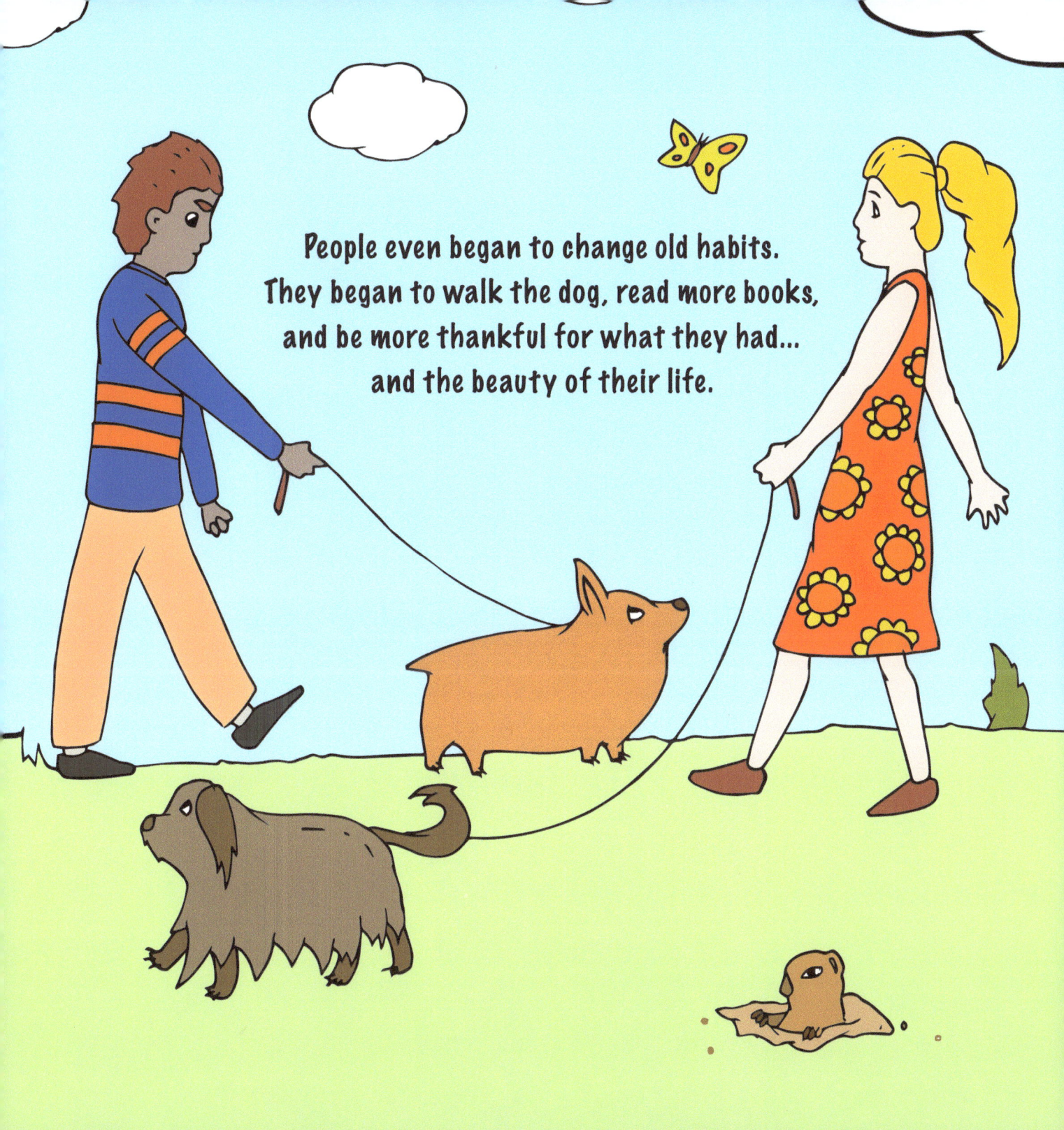

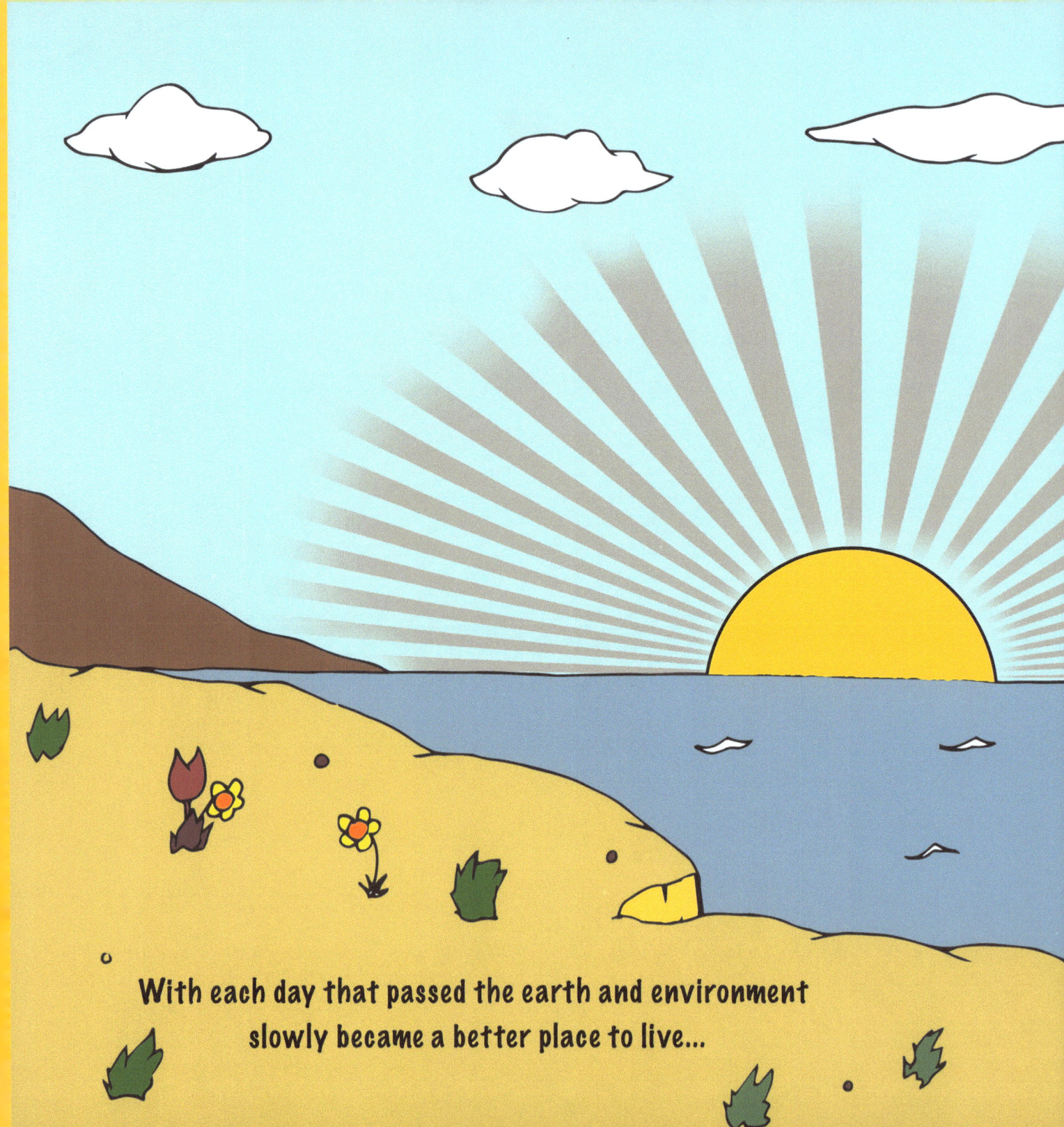

...The sky became clearer, waters in the lakes and streams became clearer, dolphins and fish returned to bays, birds sang a little louder each day, and the roads became less crowded with cars and trucks.

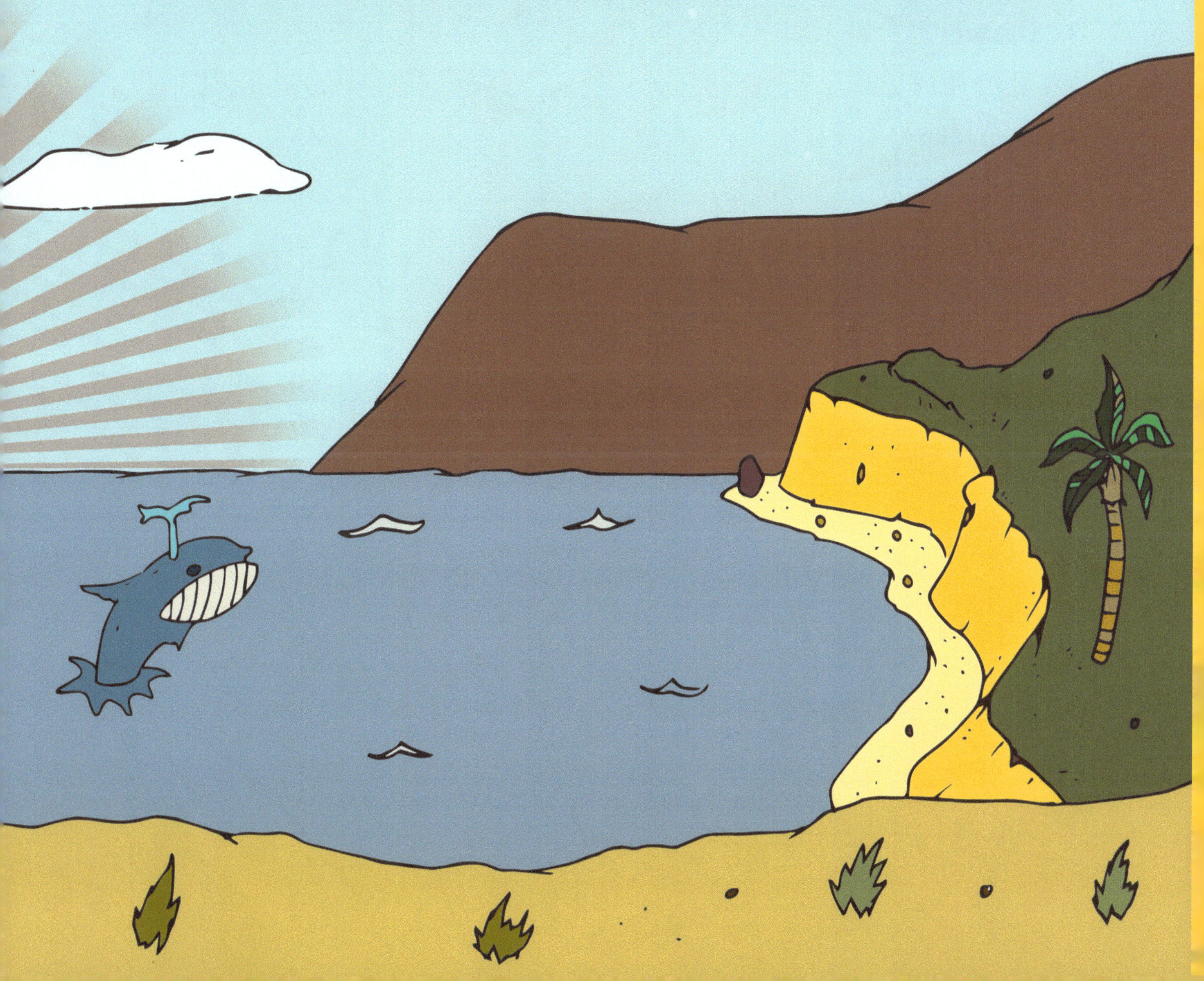

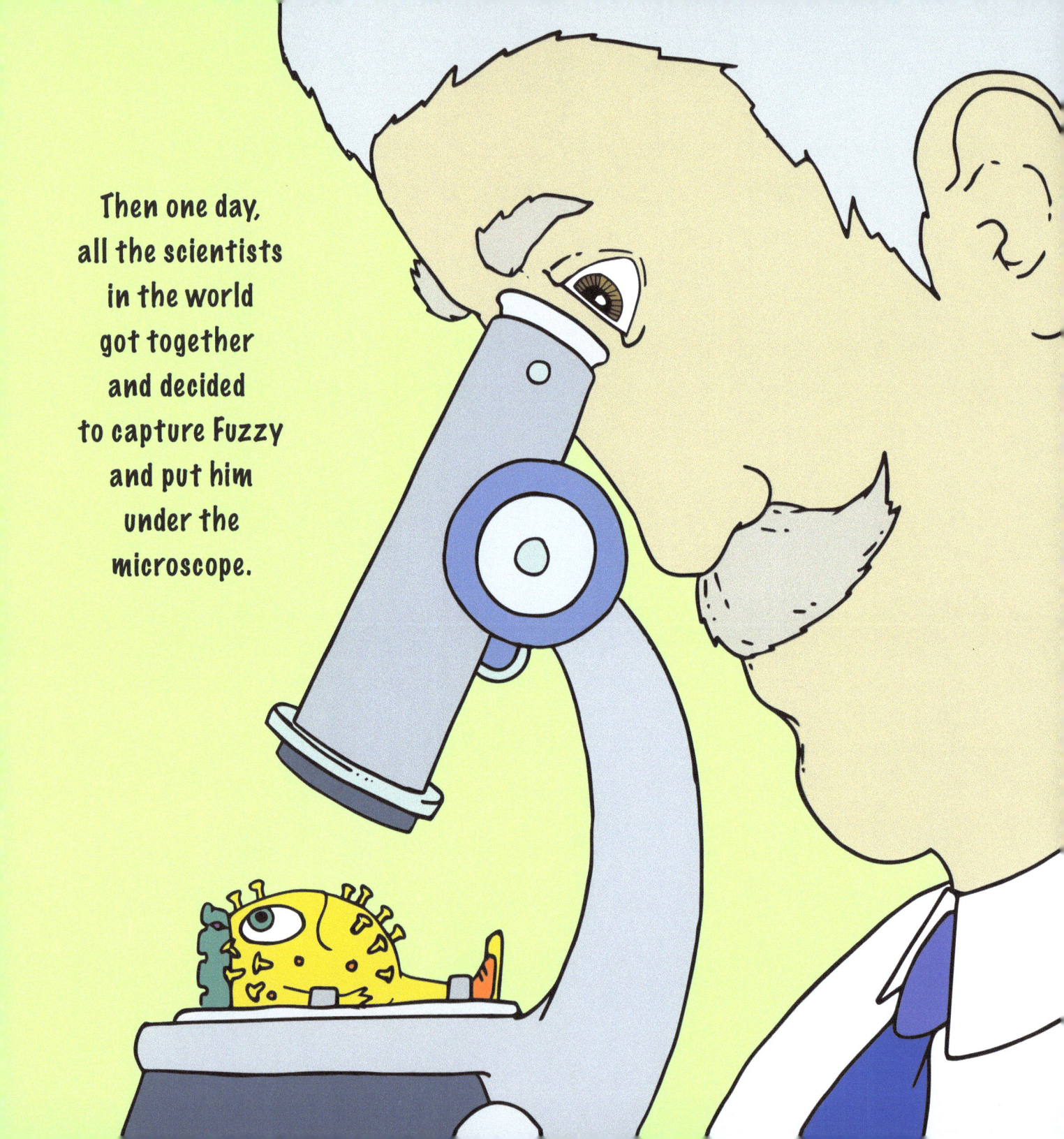

"Who is this Fuzzy the Virus?"

"How can he make the world so scared?"

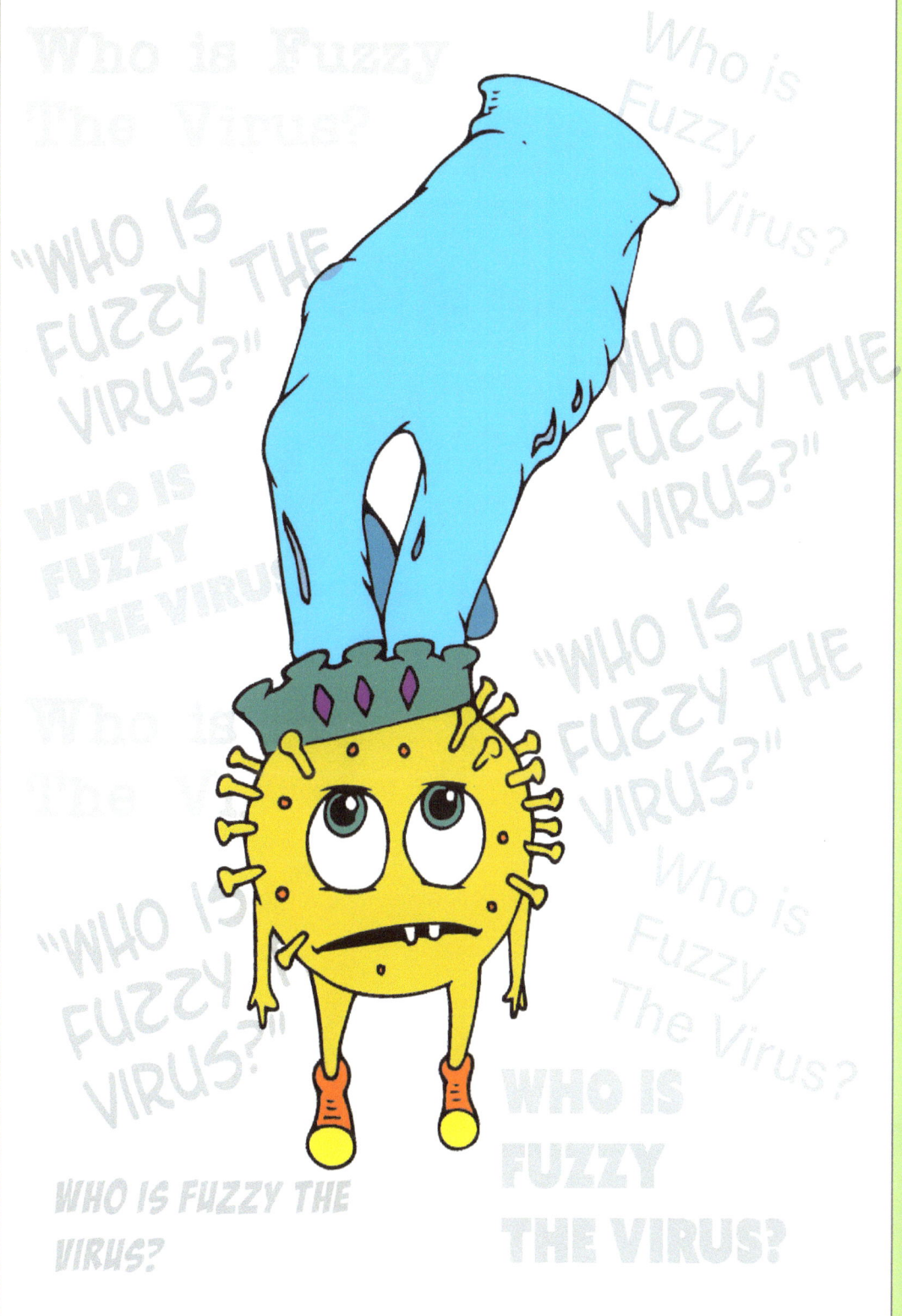

HELSINKI HOSPITAL RESULTS	BEIJING LABORATORY RESULTS	LOS ANGELES HOSPITAL RESULTS
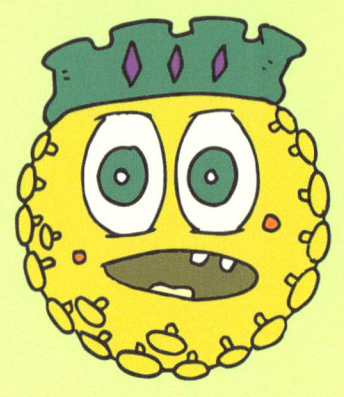	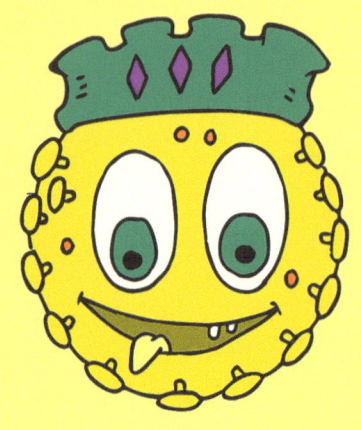	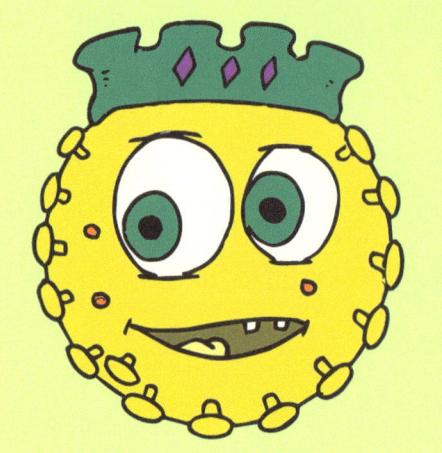
LONDON LAB CENTER RESULTS	SYDNEY SCIENCE CENTER RESULTS	RIO DE JANEIRO LAB RESULTS
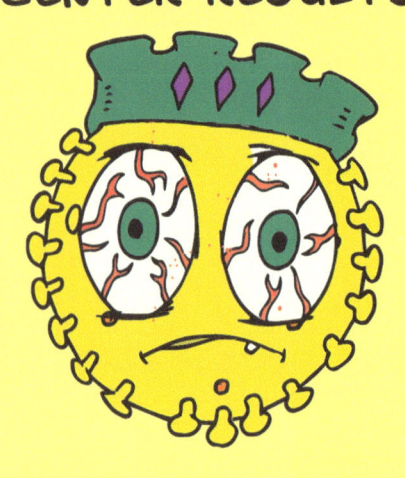	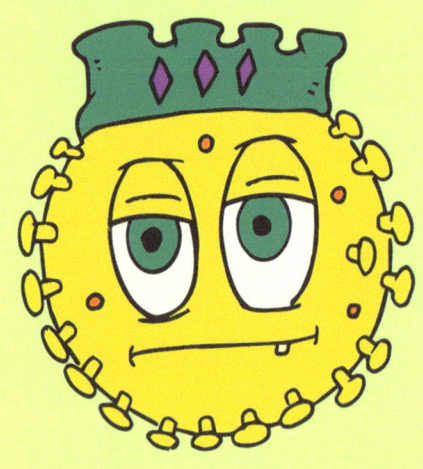	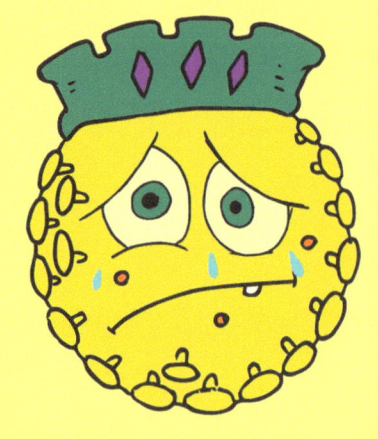

Poor little Fuzzy. Everybody wanted to know who he was. So Fuzzy was tested 1,000 different ways by all sorts of scientists, doctors, labratories and hospitals.

He was chopped, and sliced, and blended, and mixed, and poked, and probed, and tossed up and down and all around and sideways. **"WHO IS FUZZY THE VIRUS?"** That was the question everybody wanted to know.

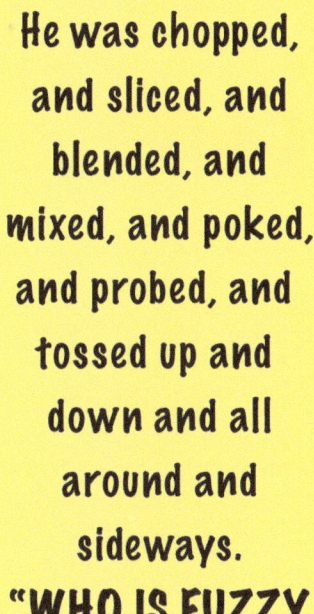

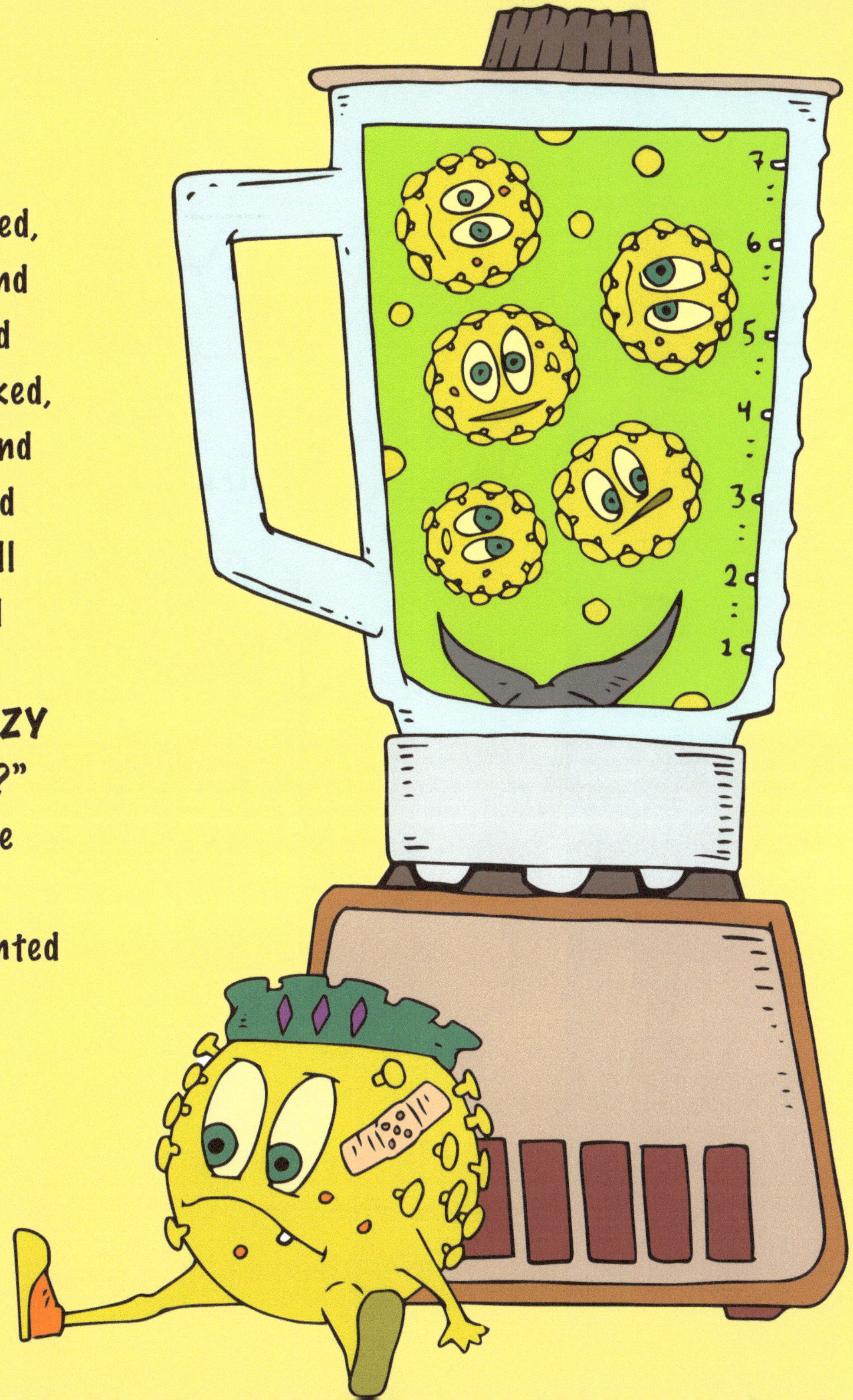

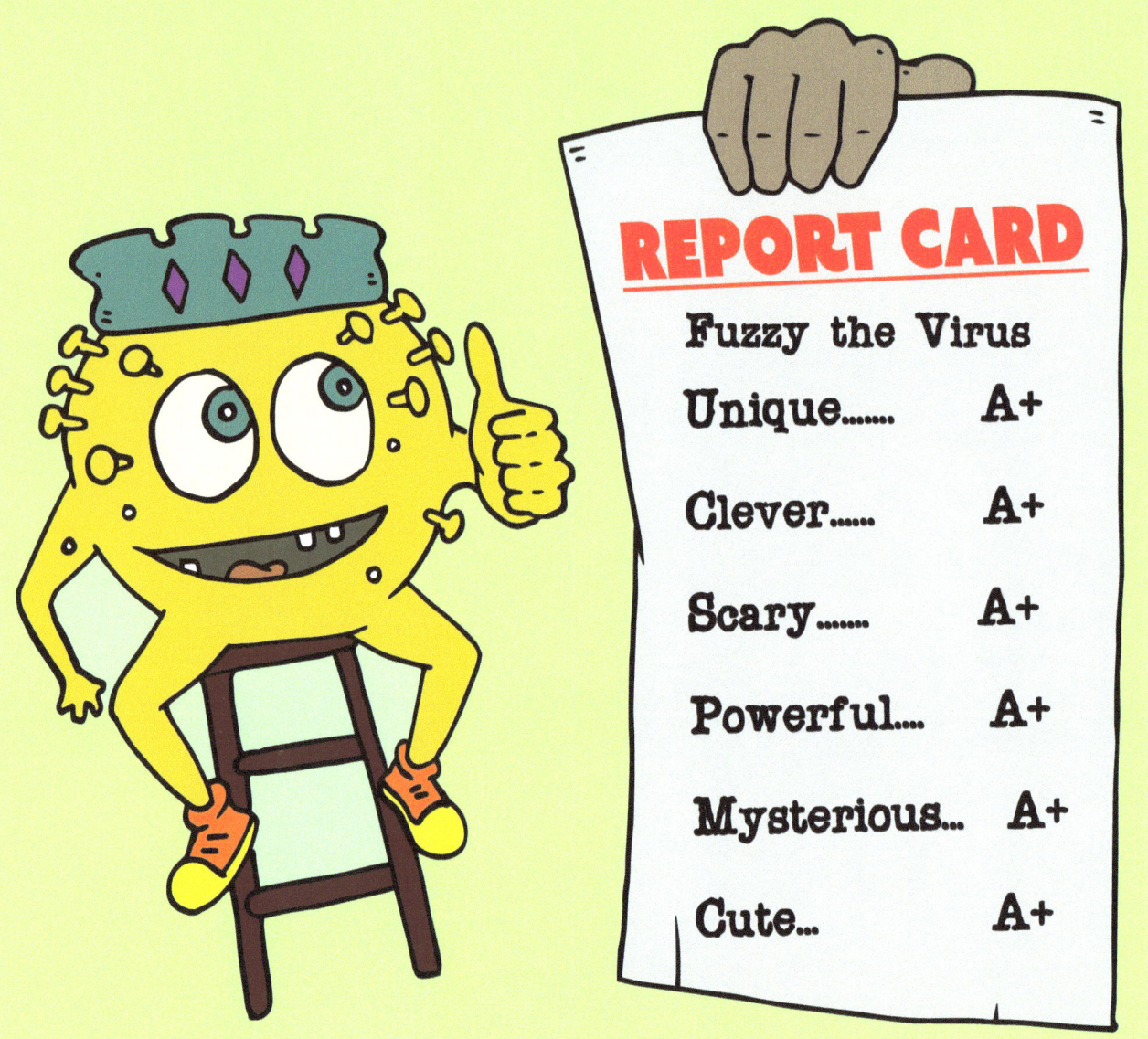

After all the tests were finished, everyone agreed...
  Fuzzy was very clever and unique, and the scientists had never seen any other virus quite like him.

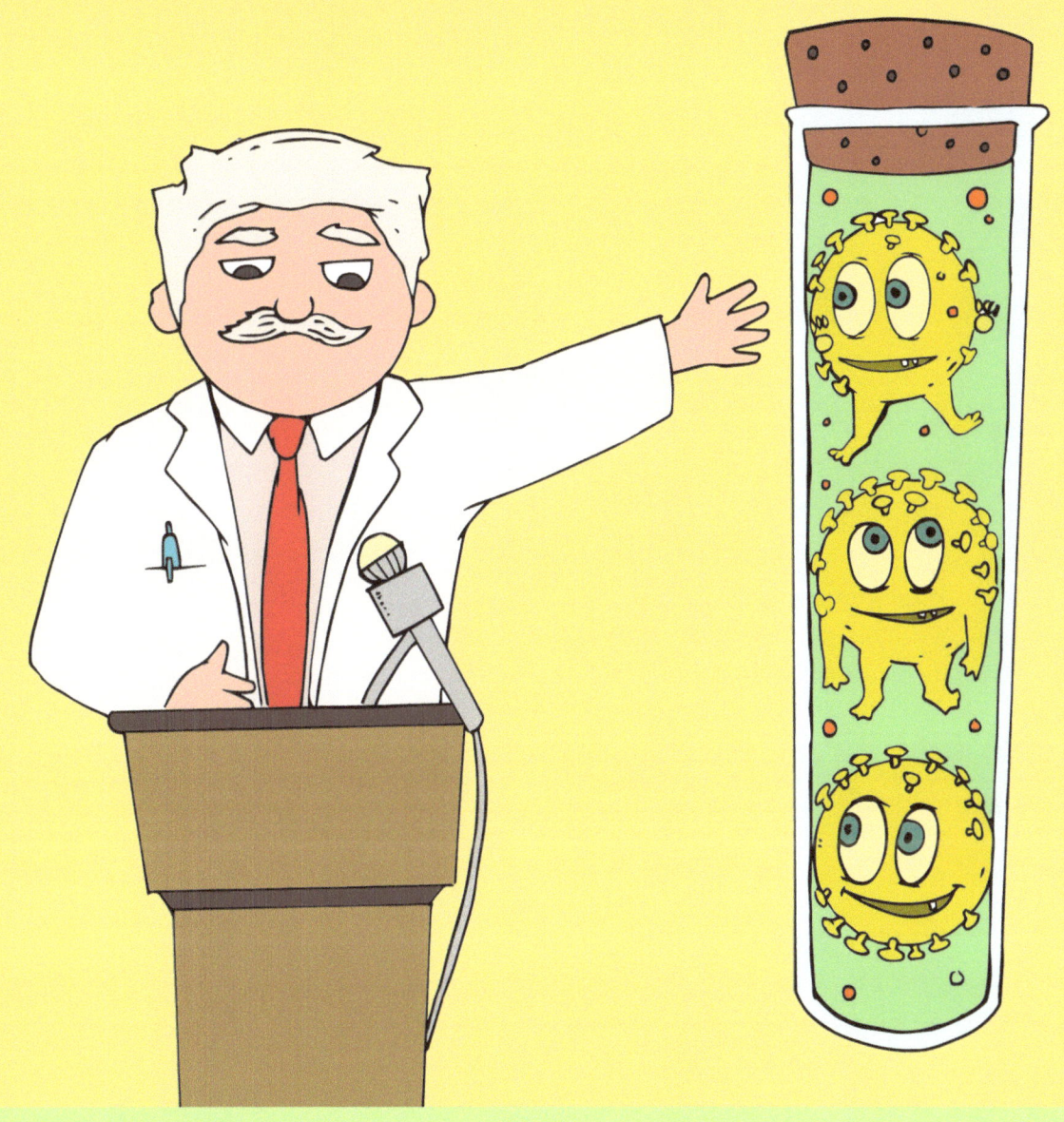

And although Fuzzy did help us all become more kind, more grateful, and helped make the world a better place to live, he was still very dangerous. "Isn't there something we can do to make him a safe friend?" everybody asked?

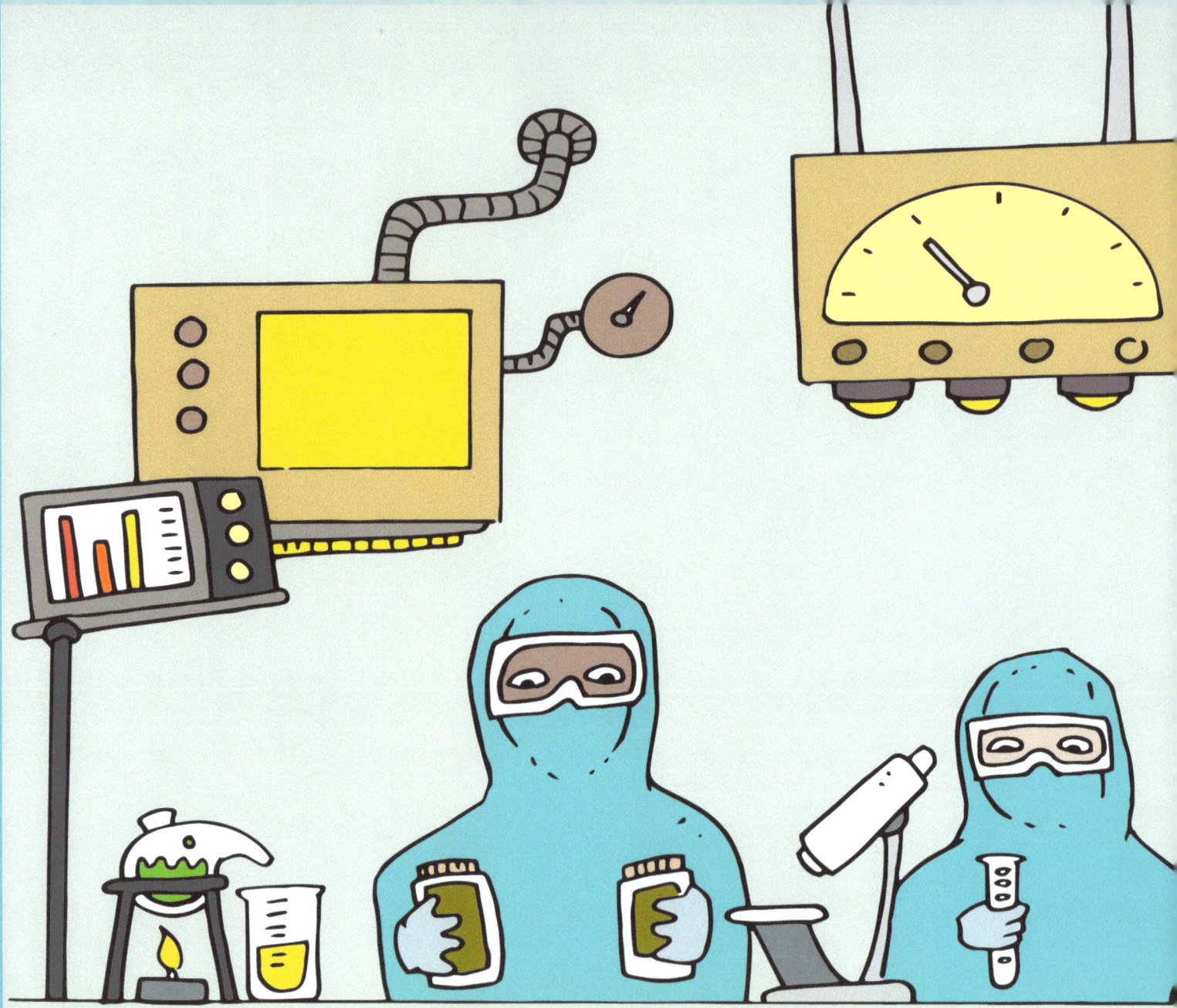

So all the scientists went back to their laboratories.
They worked day and night for months and months.

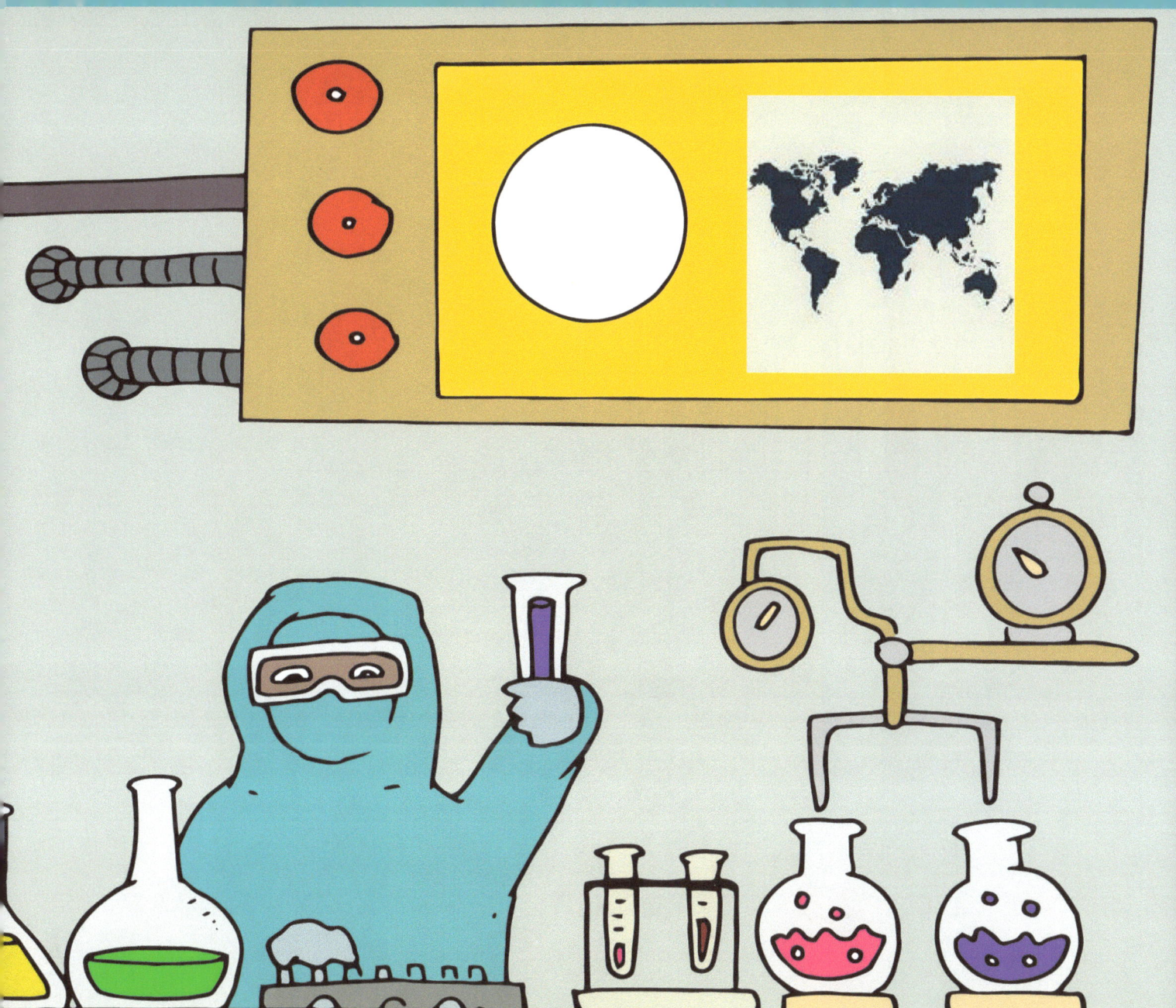

Trying to figure out a way to have Fuzzy be our friend, not our enemy... and for people not to be afraid of Fuzzy in the future.

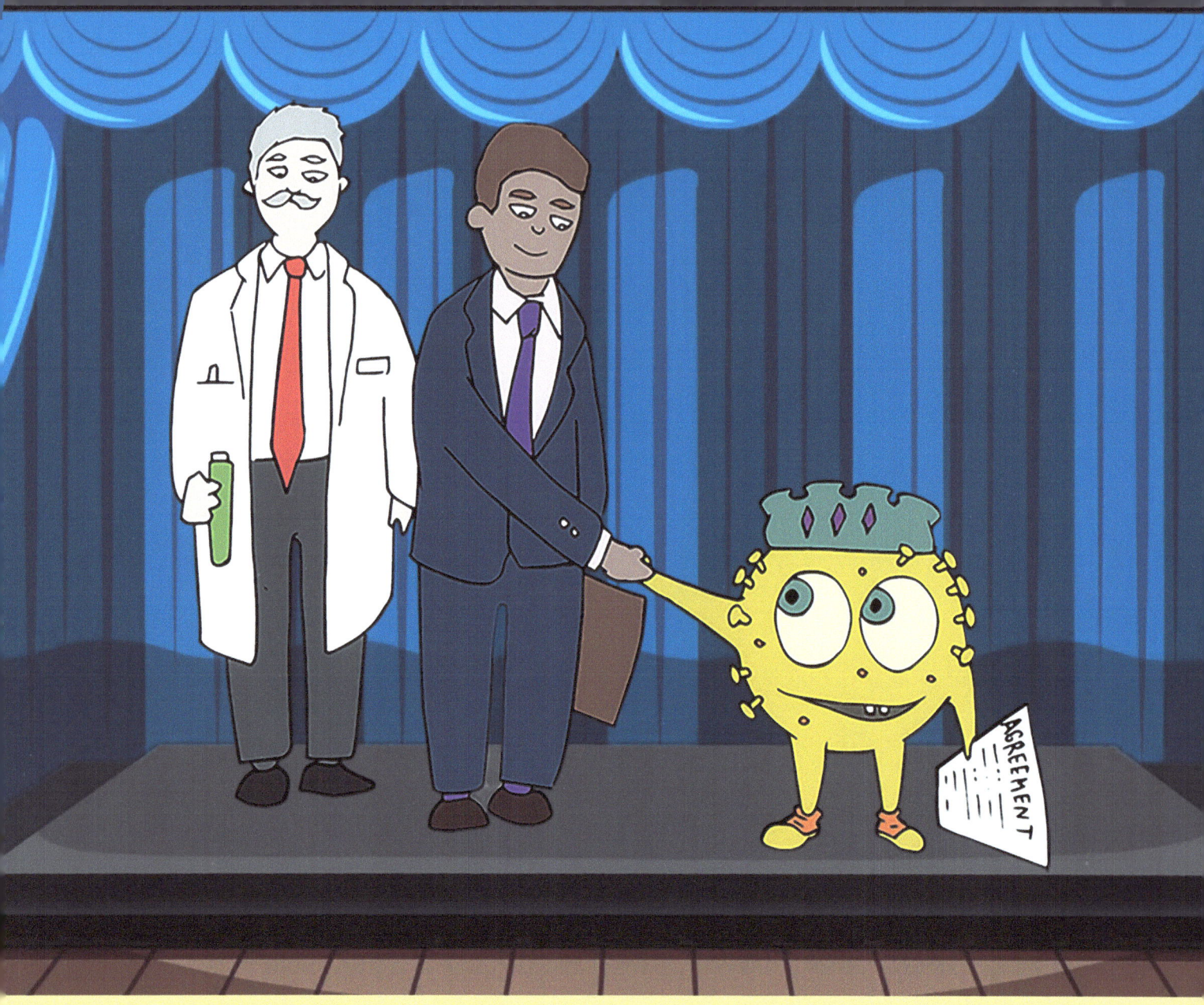

Finally, they had a good idea... and asked Fuzzy if he would help out.
Fuzzy said "YES!"

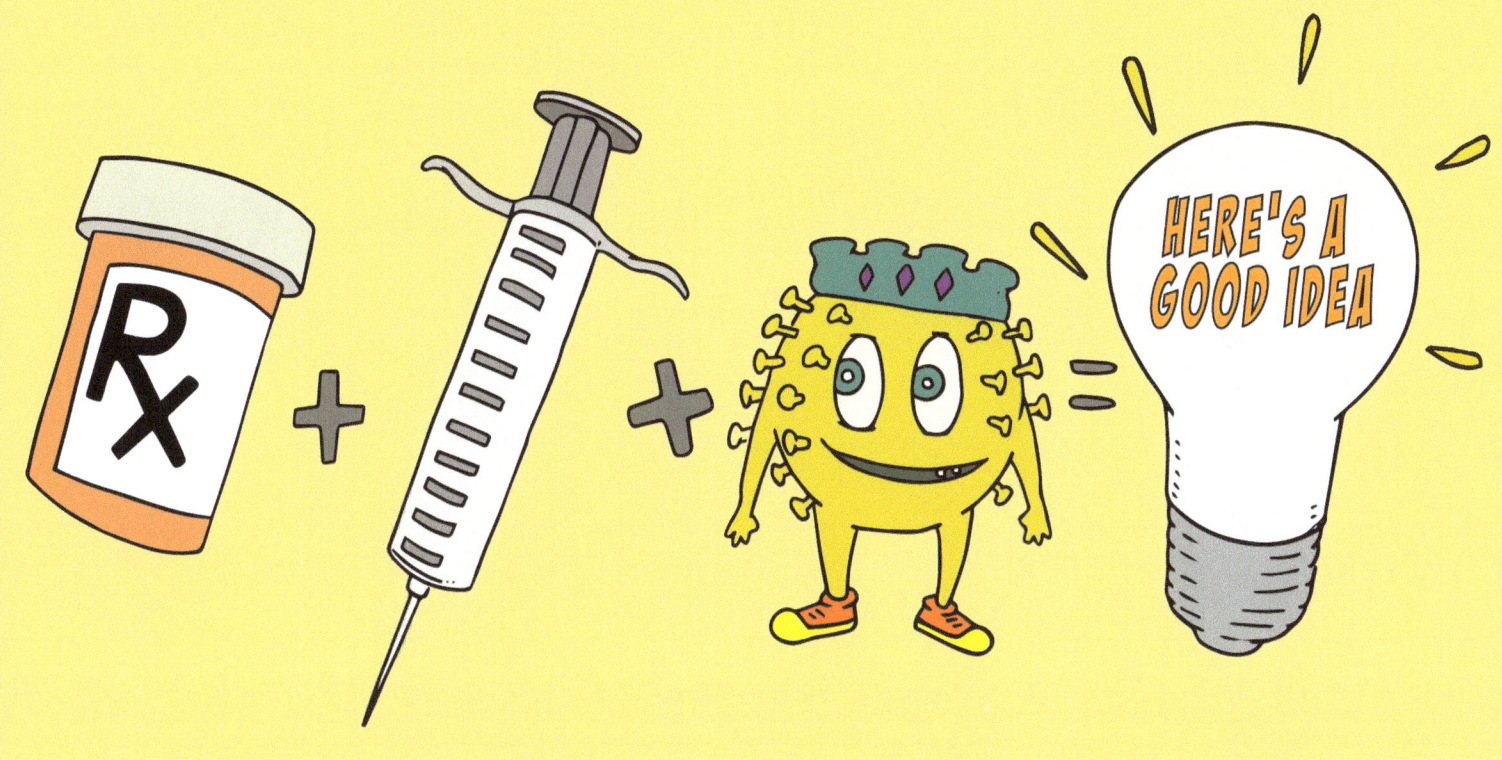

Soon, all the scientists went back to work to create a medicine that would make it safe again for Fuzzy to travel around the world, to make new friends wherever he went.

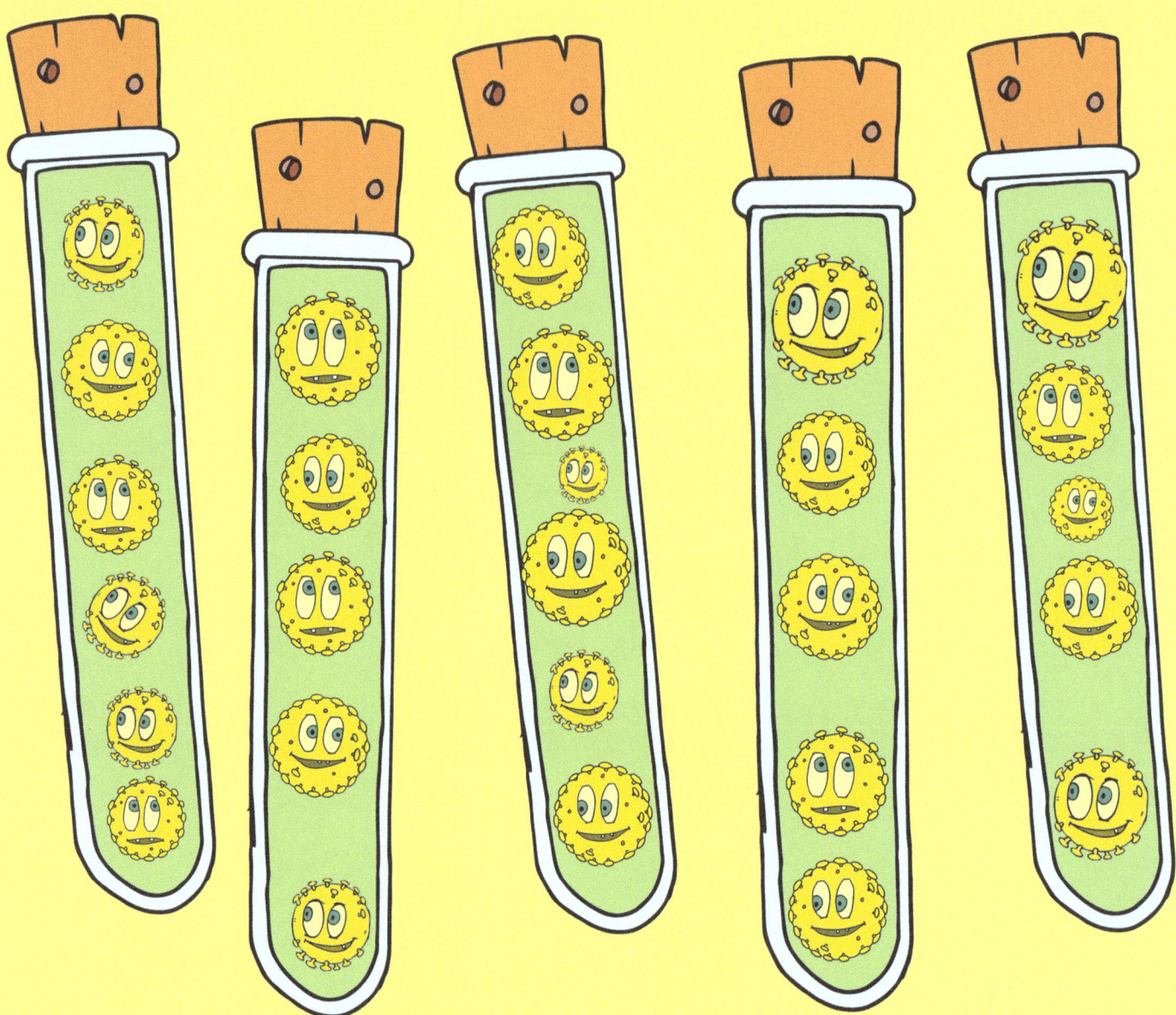

You see, what scientists found out is that Fuzzy could be our friend if there was a little Fuzzy inside each of us.

So, doctors all across the world worked hard and created a vaccine that put a very tiny little piece of Fuzzy inside every pill and shot.

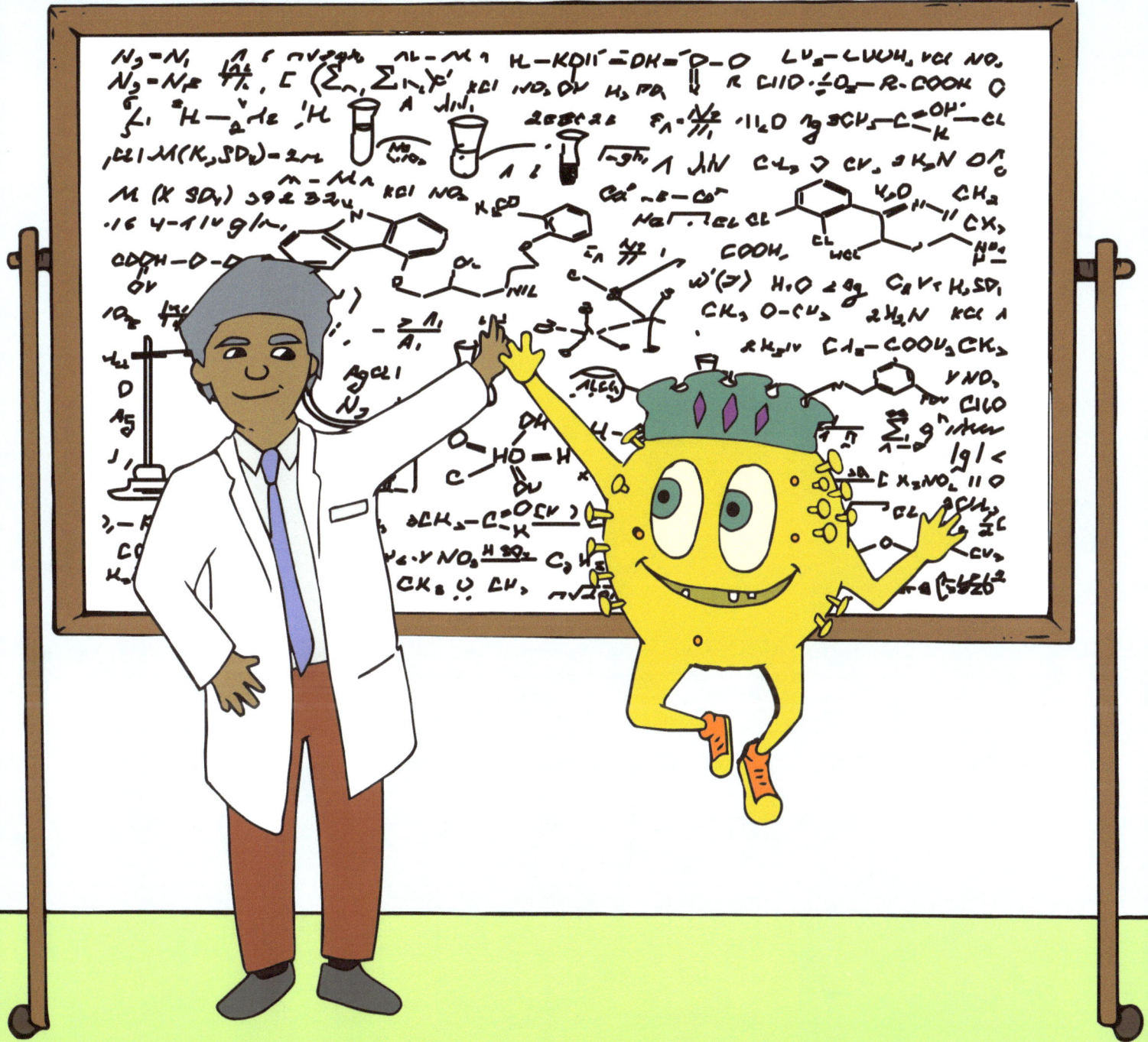

Instead of making his new friends sick, Fuzzy could now help the world be a much safer, more beautiful, and more caring place for all of us to live.

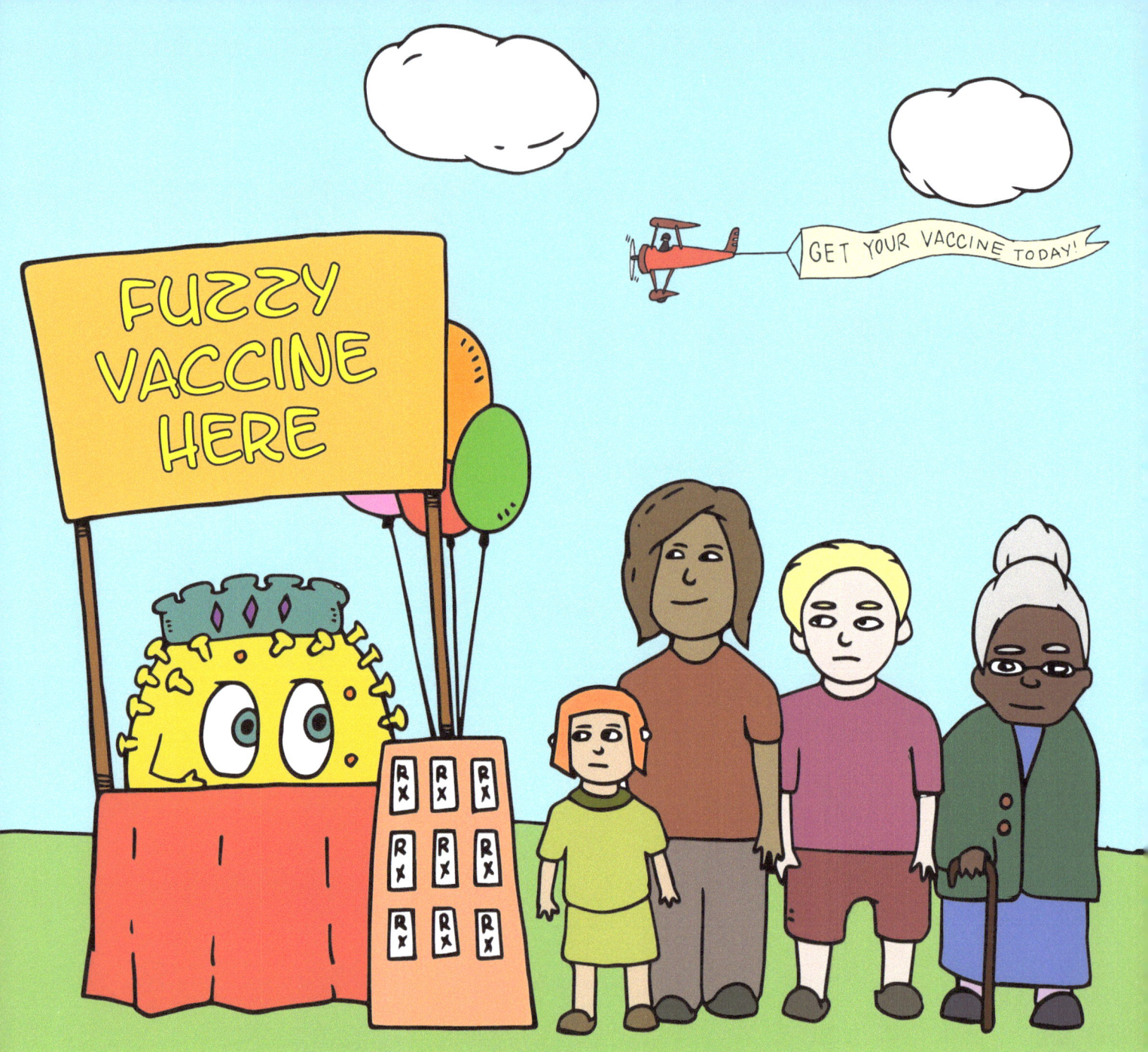

Soon, all the people began to come out of their houses and get this very special medicine.

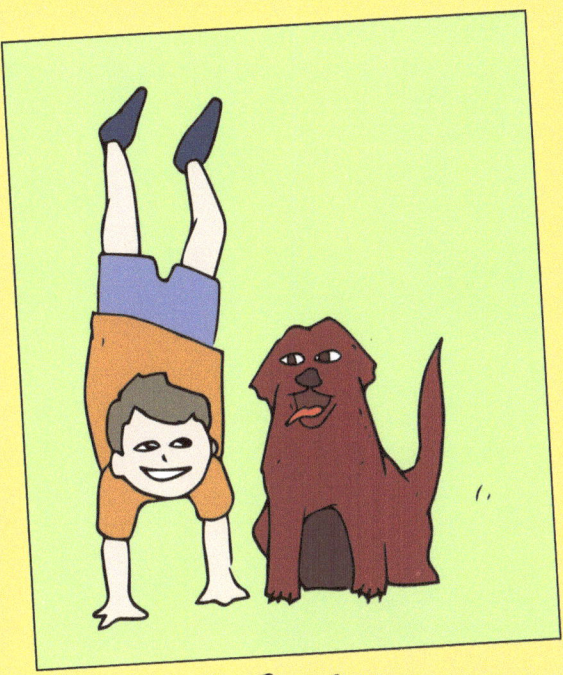
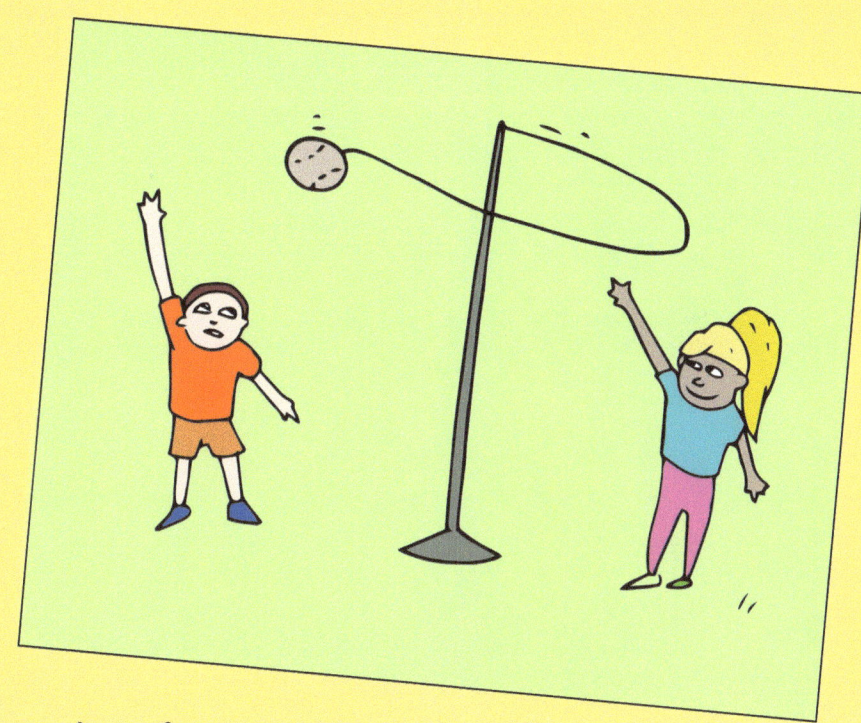

People began to go see their friends in person again,
And they began to go out to dinner again at the restaurants,
And they started to take airplane trips again,
And went back to work and back to school!

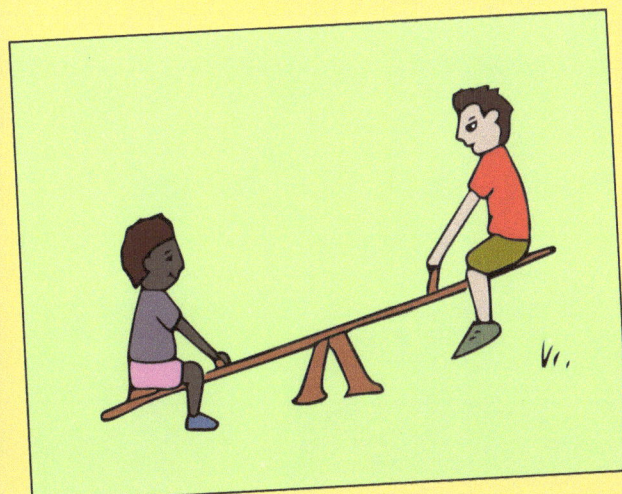
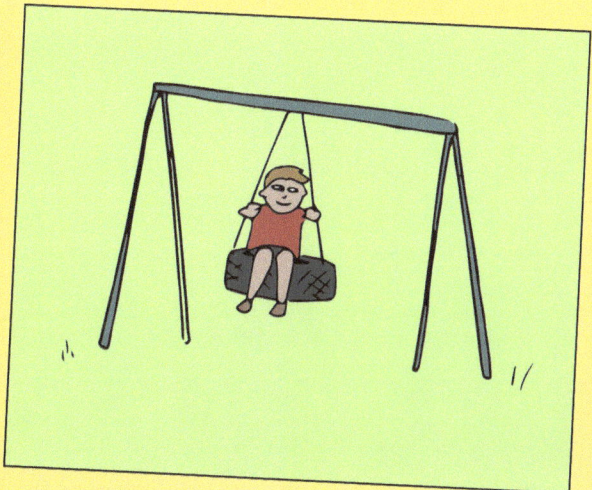

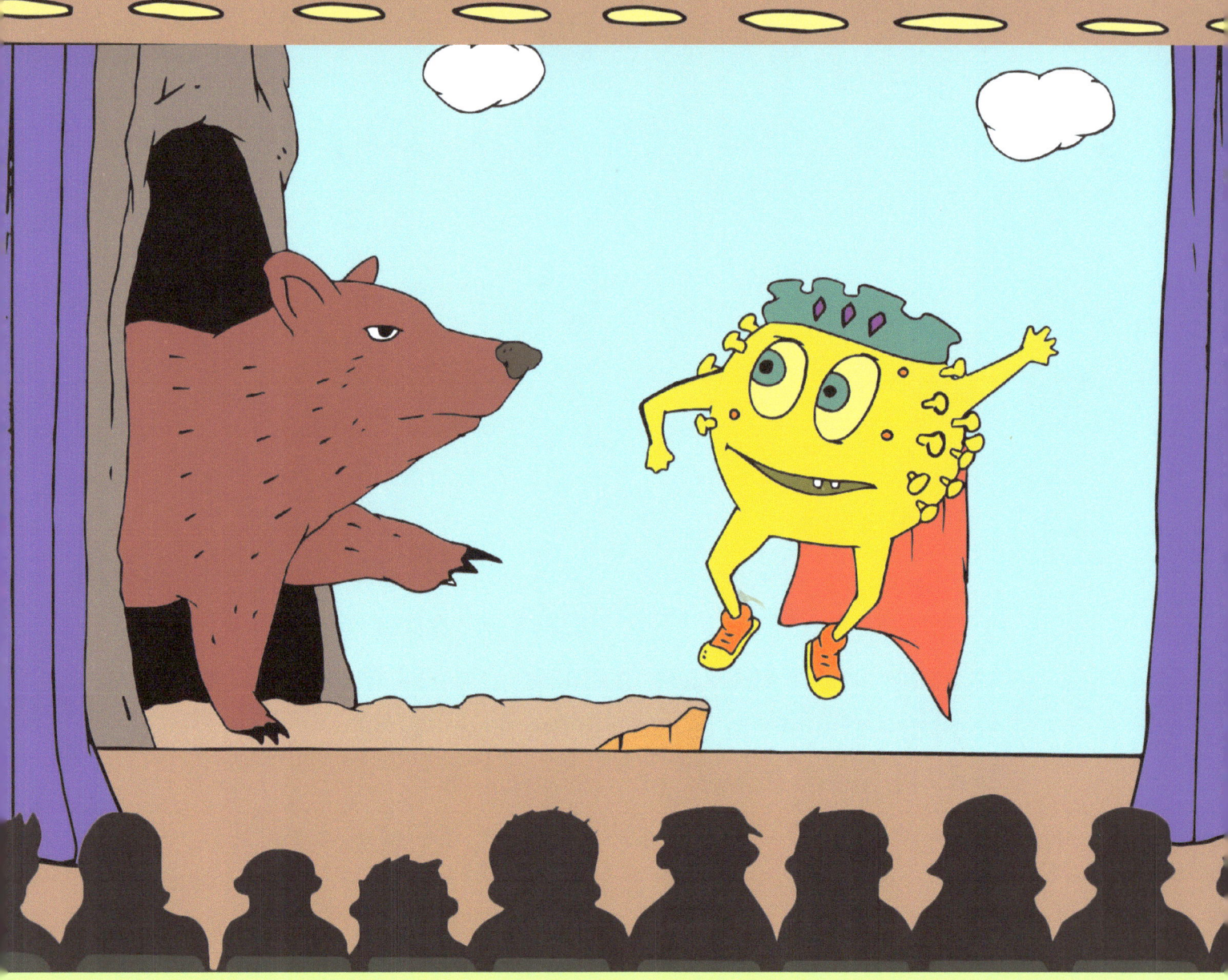

The sports teams began to play again.
Concerts and movies, high-fives and swimming, going to the beach and visiting friends and families... it all came back just like it was before everyone was scared.

Fuzzy had achieved his big dream...

He traveled and spread everywhere, becoming friends with everyone in the world.

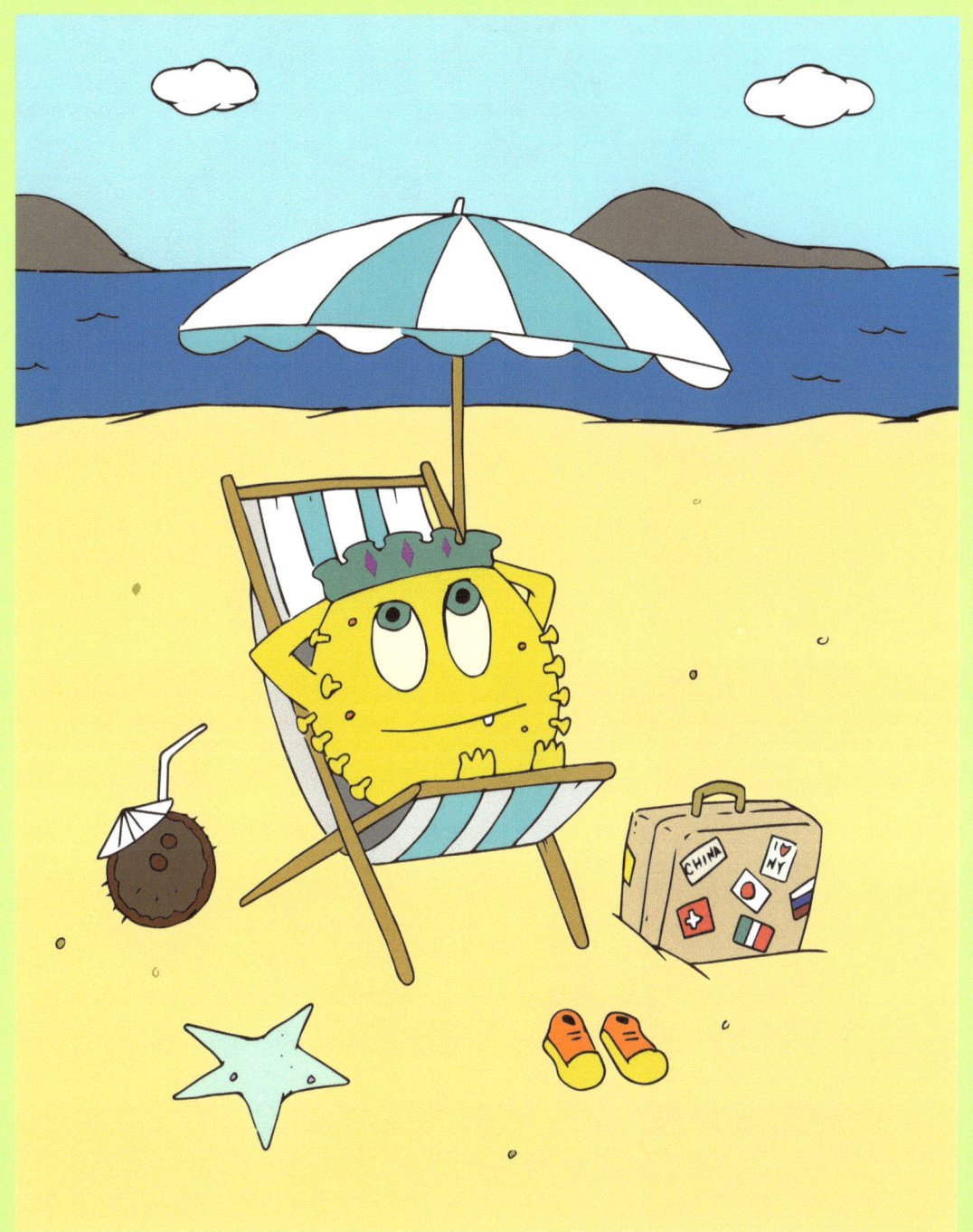

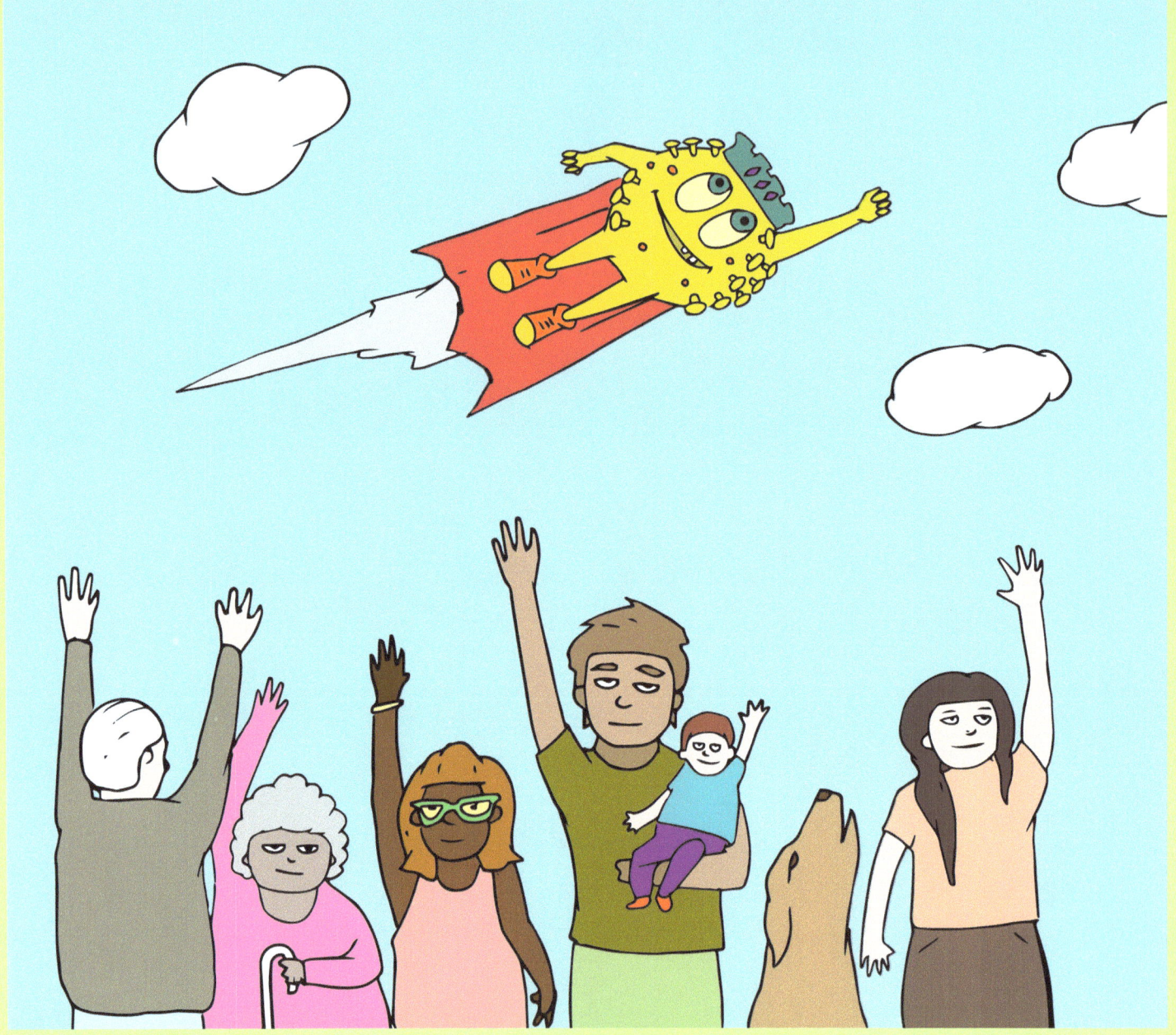

And we all learned a lot from Fuzzy the Virus.
    We learned how to live healthier...
        We learned how to overcome our fear...
            We learned how to work together in a time of need.

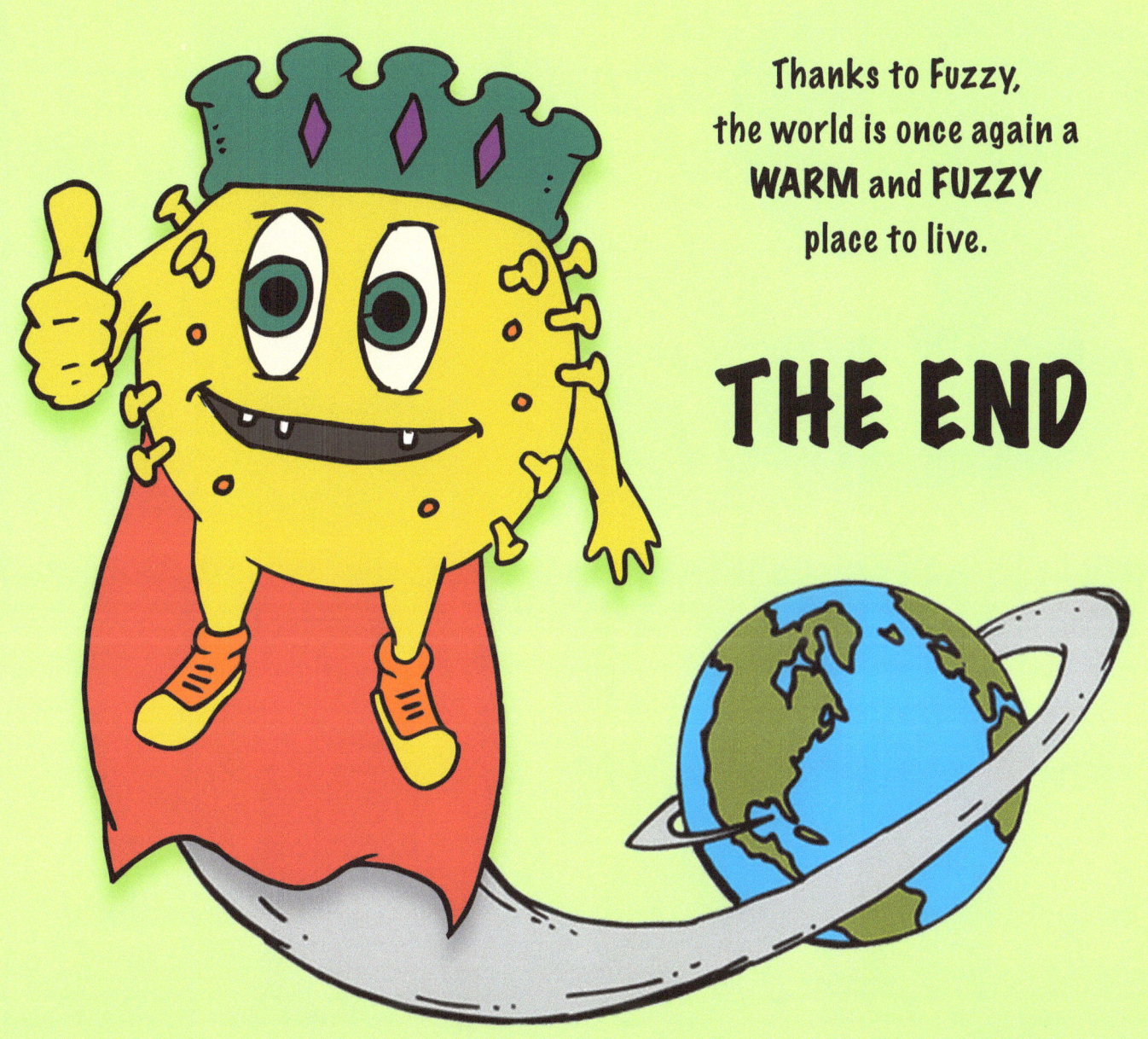

Visit Fuzzy at...

www.fuzzythevirus.com

COMING SOON...

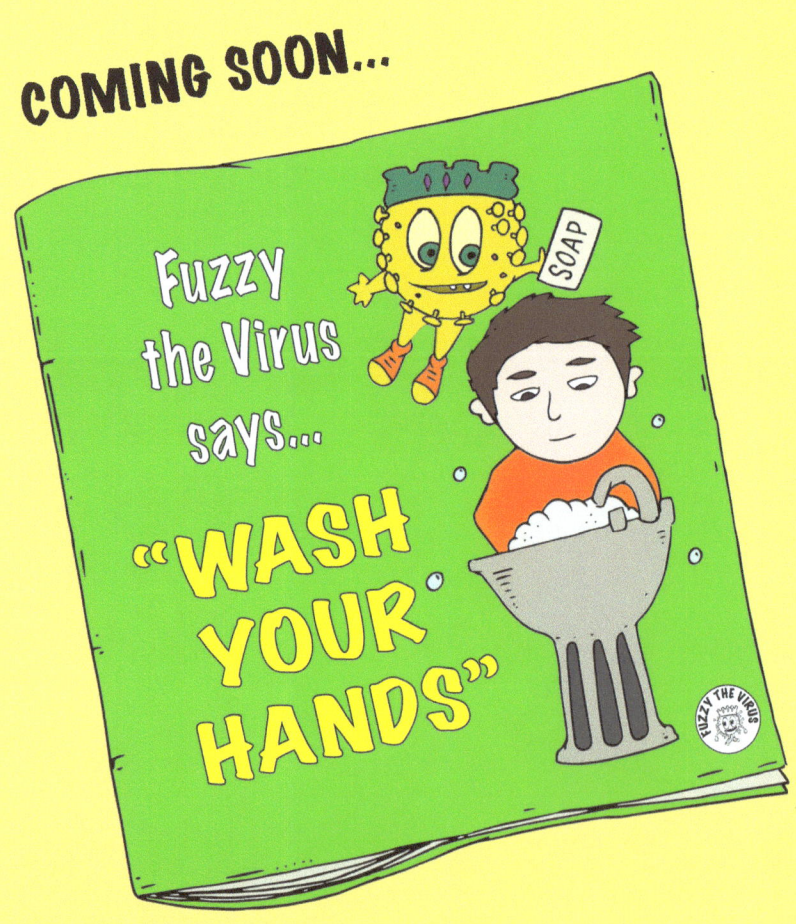

- Leave Fuzzy a book review!

- Order multiple copies (at a discount) for your office, school, friends and family!

- Order your advanced copy of Fuzzy the Virus says... "WASH YOUR HANDS!"

www.ingramcontent.com/pod-product-compliance
Lightning Source LLC
Chambersburg PA
CBHW051222220526
45473CB00003B/1136